How to survi
malpractice lawsuit

How to survive a medical malpractice lawsuit

The physician's road map for success

Ilene R. Brenner, MD
Board Certified Emergency Physician
and Adjunct Professor
Nell Hodgson School of Nursing at Emory University
Atlanta, GA, USA

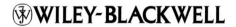

A John Wiley & Sons, Ltd., Publication

Library of Congress Cataloging-in-Publication Data
Brenner, Ilene R.
    How to survive a medical malpractice lawsuit: the physician's roadmap for success / Ilene R. Brenner.
        p.; cm.
    Includes bibliographical references and index.
    ISBN: 978-1-4443-3130-1
    1. Physicians—Malpractice. I. Title.
    [DNLM: 1. Malpractice—legislation & jurisprudence—United States. 2. Liability, Legal—United States.
3. Physicians—legislation & jurisprudence—united states. W 44 AA1 B838h 2010]
    RA1056.5.B74 2010
    610.68—dc22

                                                                                            2010002246
ISBN: 978-1-4443-3130-1

A catalogue record for this book is available from the British Library.

Set in 9.5/12pt Minion by MPS Limited, A Macmillan Company

Contents

Acknowledgments

I thank my family and friends for their support.

In particular I thank my father, Joseph Brenner, Attorney at Law, who was the Consulting Editor for this book and provided legal information.

In addition, I want to thank the following people:

Ted Pound: My personal medical malpractice defense attorney whose talent I respect and admire.

Mark Plaster: Editor of my article series in *Emergency Physician's Monthly* who got me started on this journey.

Paul S. Levine: My literary attorney.

William Sullivan, DO, JD: Helped me with a few legal topics in the book.

Valerie Clark: My personal editor and guide through the process.

Cynthia Stephenson, DO, Luis O. Vasconez, MD, and Doug Lowery-North, MD: Reviewed my manuscript and supported the project.

I want to acknowledge all the hard-working physicians who put their livelihood at risk every day they go to work, and who still practice quality medicine to the benefit of their patients despite all the obstacles in their way.

Finally, I need to thank all my patients, whose honor it has been to treat and who honor me by giving me an opportunity to be a part of their lives.

Foreword

I will never forget that thanksgiving as long as I live. We had just offered our heartfelt thanks to God for a wonderful year when the doorbell rang. To my surprise, standing at the door in a blinding storm was a deputy sheriff. I thought, what would bring you out on a night like this? There must have been a burglary in the neighborhood. Then he handed me the letter, shook his head, and said, "I'm really sorry doctor to do this to you on Thanksgiving. It's just my job." I did not understand his apology until I saw the return address on the letter. It was a law firm. And I was being sued. I returned to the table and tried to act as if it was nothing. But I could not eat. My whole world, as well as my stomach, was turned upside down.

Every physician who has ever been sued, and that is most of us, knows that feeling of loss, frustration, and bewilderment. It is in that moment that you want someone to help you, to give you some practical advice, to hold your hand. Ilene Brenner has done just that in a professional way with a very personal approach.

There are quite a number of books on how to avoid getting sued. Some will help you to be a better clinician, improve your documentation, and communicate more effectively; all skills that will lower your chances of ever being sued. But as most of us know, litigation, like lightening, can never be predicted very accurately. You practice the best medicine you know how. You document your charts with compulsive detail. You treat your patients like they are your own family. But then something happens, and there is a bad outcome. And the patient looks around for someone to blame and you get sued. Then the question becomes, what do you do when lightening strikes?

As the editor-in-chief of *Emergency Physician's Monthly*, a publication read by over 40,000 emergency physicians across the nation, I work constantly, in various ways to help emergency physicians avoid litigation, prepare for litigation, and to recover from litigation. I have been on both sides of the fence. In addition to being a physician, I am also an attorney and the former medical legal editor of *Emergency Department Law*. I have been sued, and I have helped prepare fellow physicians to defend themselves. So when

I read the first submission of Dr. Brenner on the topic of *How to Survive a Malpractice Suit*, it was clear that she knew what she was talking about. Her style was at once very intimate and personal. She gains your confidence with her honesty. Then she walks you through the practical steps that you needed to take to properly defend yourself, your practice, your property, and your sense of self. Her advice is not just personal, it is very practical.

The financial burden of medical malpractice lawsuits is well known to most Americans, especially those of us who are the targets of that litigation. Fear of being sued is the number one cause of over testing and over treating patients and may account for, in the estimate of some economists, up to a quarter of our nation's overall healthcare spending. Furthermore, although physicians win the overwhelming majority of cases brought against them, as the amounts of awards have skyrocketed, insurance premiums have risen as well, driving many physicians out of practice. The financial burden of litigation is felt throughout the system. But what about the impact on the physicians themselves?

Once named in a suit, even if you are only peripherally involved, it may take years to clear your name or resolve the suit. In the interim, they do not know how, let alone if, they will survive. Lawyers representing their physician clients do not have or do not take the time to hold their clients by the hand. Maybe it is the natural aversion of doctors for lawyers and vice versa. Whatever, it just does not happen very often. The physicians feel left alone with no one who understands them, no one to answer the detail questions about how, when, where, and sometimes even why. That is when you really wish you had a malpractice defense lawyer in the family. Dr. Brenner did.

When Dr. Brenner was served with a suit for medical negligence, in addition to her legal counsel, she turned to a trusted friend, her father, who just happened to be a seasoned medical malpractice trial attorney. Between her paid counsel and her "family lawyer," she was able to get answers for the little detail questions that get overlooked and only thought of after the appointment with your attorney. Moreover, she was able to ask about the nuance of the personal side of litigation. The combination made for an intimate yet useful guide.

When it is all said and done, no one can completely prevent a physician from exposure to malpractice litigation. Bad outcomes occur. We may even ask ourselves whether we would have taken a different course had we been able to see the future. Moreover, nothing can insulate a physician from the shock of being sued by the one you attempted to help. But when it does occur, it is really useful to have a guide who can walk you through the experience. Dr. Brenner offers practical advice in a way that allows you to trust her. The wise person will take the advice and be better prepared to weather the storm.

Mark Plaster, MD, JD

Introduction

Approximately 80 billion dollars are spent every year by physicians as a result of their practice of defensive medicine. They order extra tests, do additional procedures, and prescribe superfluous antibiotics. Why would well-trained physicians practice this way? They are hoping that their thoroughness will stave off any potential lawsuits.

For most physicians, medicine is more than a vocation; it is a calling. These highly intelligent people sacrifice the best years of their lives to work 100+ hour weeks at less than minimum wage. Most doctors would tell you that the reason they decided to go through all this time and trouble, at extreme sacrifice on both personal and financial levels, was out of an idealistic intent to help sick people become well.

Having a multiyear apprenticeship in residency training does create physicians who are both competent and confident in their practice of medicine. However, with board certification and yearly re-certifications, on top of the required continuing medical education (CME) courses, and reading scores of articles and journals, the training never really ends.

In fact, the core identity of most physicians is indelibly imprinted with the field of medicine. Unlike many other professions where people can leave their job at work, a doctor is always a doctor (any physician who has answered the call at a restaurant or on an airplane knows exactly what I mean). It is for this reason that physicians are uniquely vulnerable to a medical malpractice lawsuit; in both a literal and a psychological sense.

The long road to become a physician prevents most from getting expertise that would enable them to seek another vocation; few have the skill set to even work as a secretary. And fewer have the ability to work in another career where they could earn a salary commensurate with their current income. Physicians have committed their lives, and their livelihood, to the practice of medicine. When something like a lawsuit threatens to derail their future in the only profession in which they have skills and passion, they panic; which is understandable since an unfavorable result can do irreparable harm to their career.

Every doctor seeks to avoid getting sued, but few doctors know what to do once it happens. Risk management courses abound, but they are not mandatory and relatively few doctors attend. Despite the information in these courses, there is still a surprising dearth of information when it comes to what happens AFTER you get sued.

Although doctors spend years in learning the language of medicine, few have any familiarity with the legal profession beyond what they see on television. A very small percentage of the education of physicians includes the legal aspects of medicine. Much of these hours are dedicated to government regulations such as EMTALA and HIPAA, and the defensive practice of medicine. Little if any attention is given to the legal process in a medical malpractice lawsuit. And this is why, when first served with papers declaring a complaint against them by one of their patients, physicians are completely unprepared for the crucial moments that follow.

Fortunately for me, I won my case in a jury trial, and I learned many lessons as a result. During my journey through the legal system, I had an excellent resource to draw from: my father, who is a defendant medical malpractice trial attorney. Shortly after winning, a number of my friends were sued as well. They asked me a myriad of similar questions. I shared with them the knowledge I obtained through my experience, my attorney, and information gleaned from years of assisting my father on his cases. It occurred to me that if these intelligent physicians were all requiring the same advice, lots of other physicians likely needed it as well.

This inspired me to write an article entitled, *OK, so you've been sued. Now what?*, which was published by *Emergency Physician's Monthly Magazine* in 2007. That first article was the beginning of a series of articles about medical malpractice.

The extremely positive responses I received spurred me on to expand my readership beyond emergency physicians. Certainly, all medical professionals can benefit from advice about what is considered one of the most stressful events in a physician's life: being sued for medical malpractice.

I have consolidated and expanded upon my articles into a book that I hope will arm the physicians with knowledge that will help them best navigate their way through the arduous legal process.

The average physician heads into the legal arena totally unprepared for what is to follow. For the uninformed, the experience can not only be frightening but also be career ending. It is my belief that my book will help prepare physicians for battle. It is imperative that physicians be active participants in their case. Doctors cannot sit back and assume that their attorney will save them. They have to save themselves.

What is included in this book?

This book is divided into several chapters covering the time period that begins with the moment you receive your summons. It walks the reader through every aspect of the lawsuit, including the posttrial appeal.

You will also find additional mock deposition testimony examples than that were present in my series of articles. In addition, there are specific examples to help assist you in your cross-examination.

There is a chapter on the psychology of a medical malpractice lawsuit, which details the complex and emotional aspects of litigation. The final chapter of Section 1 is entitled, *What if you lose?* The possibility of an appeal means that there is still hope.

Section 2 of the book provides tips on lawsuit prevention. Of course, nobody can prevent a lawsuit, but there are some things that can be done that will minimize the risk, or at least help your case should you be sued. Important issues such as informed consent and risk management are discussed.

There is no specific legal advice given in this book. Although I have consulted with attorneys in writing this book, I am not an attorney, and I make no claims to be an authority on legal issues. For that, I recommend speaking with a medical malpractice attorney in your state.

Although I am a physician, I am not attempting to give any advice on the practice of medicine. I cannot guarantee that following the information in this book will lead to a positive result in your lawsuit. I do, however, believe that it will dramatically improve your chances.

I hope that no one needs to utilize any of this guidance. Unfortunately, statistically, most of us will. It is not a sign of weakness to be involved in a lawsuit. In fact, it is a badge of honor that you made it through the legal system with your sanity intact.

People sue for various reasons: unreasonably high expectations, desire for a monetary reward, revenge for feeling condescended to, and because other physicians convinced them that they were victims of medical malpractice. Being sued does not make you a bad doctor. Making mistakes does not make you a bad doctor either. It makes you human.

So if you have been sued, do not wallow in confusion and self-pity. Take charge. The following chapter tells you how.

Section 1   **The long road to trial**

Chapter 1 **You've been served! Now what?**

That dreaded day arrives. And no it is not just a bad dream. That police officer at your front door is not ringing the doorbell to warn you of a prowler in the neighborhood. He has come to serve you with papers notifying you of a complaint filed by a patient: a patient you may or may not remember seeing. Although anybody who serves you with papers is called a process server, in some jurisdictions, like mine, it is done by a sheriff's deputy.

The feeling is akin to being hit on the head with a bat, stabbed in the back, and disemboweled, all at the same time. Thoughts run through your mind like, "Will I lose my job?"; "Is my money protected?"; "Am I a bad doctor?"; and "Is my career over?"

You are justifiably depressed, confused, frustrated, and angry. When you have had a few minutes, hours, or days to assimilate this experience that unfortunately has begun a new chapter in your life, you undoubtedly ask, "Now what?"

When it happened to me, I called my father. Then again, not everyone has a medical malpractice defense trial attorney for a father. Most physicians do not have an attorney who is readily available to give appropriate and timely advice to initiate damage control. Through this book I am going to suggest what to do and, equally important, what not to do.

FIRST: Obtain a copy of your medical malpractice policy and make sure you can answer the following questions

Most of us think paying out an exorbitant sum of money every year is the extent of our necessary knowledge of the policy. But there are a few things you should know about your policy, and if you do not know, you should find out soon.

How to Survive a Medical Malpractice Lawsuit. By © Ilene R. Brenner. Published 2010 Blackwell Publishing.

> Some key clauses to know:
> **1** Policy limits
> **2** Ability to choose an attorney
> **3** If you have the right to refuse settlement

Q1. What are my policy limits?

This is especially important in states that do not have caps on noneconomic damages such as pain and suffering. If the patient's economic damages are likely to relatively low, and you have caps limiting the noneconomic component, then your typical one million dollar policy limit will more than suffice. You can rest easy because you will not become destitute if you lose. (For more information about damages, see Chapters 2 and 9.)

Also, if this is a high economic damages case, for example, a patient with a long stay in the intensive care unit, loss of wages, disability, and loss of future income, you will know if you are adequately or inadequately covered in the event that you lose. If you are not adequately covered, you may want to consider settling the case to protect your personal assets. (For more information on settlements, see Chapter 8, *Should you settle?*)

I am told by a number of medical malpractice attorneys that it is rare for plaintiff attorneys to pursue a physician's personal assets when their limits are exceeded by a high verdict. However, it is still possible, and if you have not yet been sued, now is the time you should review your limits. Also, review your asset protection plan. But I am not sure if that actually works, because a ruthless plaintiff's attorney may find a loophole that allows them access to your money.

Q2. Do I get to choose an attorney or must I accept whoever is assigned? Is there a pool of attorneys from which I can choose?

This is important if you know of a good attorney that you want to request. Also, plaintiffs often sue multiple doctors, including your employer. Sometimes your employer will "assign" you the same attorney as they have. This can pose a conflict of interest if your attorney is representing both of you, often to your detriment. (See more about this topic in Chapter 3, *What is a conflict of interest and how do I resolve one?*)

If you feel that you do have a conflict of interest with your codefendants and can request a separate attorney, do so. (For more information on choosing an attorney, see Chapter 3, *How to choose your attorney.*)

In general, the process of picking a law firm to represent you should involve colleague recommendations, peer reputation, and insurance company suggestions.

The insurance company will have to retain an attorney for you to respond to the complaint quickly relatively soon, because, depending on the jurisdiction, you may have as few as 20 days from the day you were served with the papers to submit a response.

However, some policies give you the right to select an attorney. If you already have a relationship with an attorney on the insurance company's panel (of defense attorneys acceptable to the insurance company), you can request that law firm to represent you.

Often, you are not told that you have a choice even when your policy says you do, and the insurance company will assign you an attorney without asking your opinion of their selection. You need to ask questions and make it clear that you will be a proactive client. You need to know your rights.

If you do not have any ability to choose an attorney in your policy, then you can expect to be assigned an attorney. When you accept someone that the insurance company approves of, they will pay for the attorney's fees. You could insist on hiring your own attorney at your own expense to protect your interests if you do not approve of the choices offered to you (see Chapter 3 for more information). However, you do have an insurance policy that is actually a contract. You must accept the terms of the contract if you expect them to cover you for any judgments. Although you could hire private counsel to work with your assigned attorney, this is usually not necessary. They cannot try your case for you, but they can protect your interests by keeping abreast of developments in the case that you would otherwise be unaware of and give you advice to help optimize the precarious situations between codefendants.

Insurance companies' goal is to minimize losses. It is in their best interest to have excellent qualified counsel. Therefore, any law firm approved by the insurance company should be more than capable. If you do not like the attorney assigned to your case, you do have options beyond hiring private counsel. I detail these options in Chapter 3.

Too often, the shock of a lawsuit turns previously confident, curious physicians into passive-aggressive clients who wait for the insurance company to make decisions for them. This approach is potentially dangerous. You have to look out for your own interests.

Q3. Do I have the right to refuse settlement?
It may not seem like a big deal, but nowadays even a low settlement is considered a loss as it raises your risk status with the insurance company.

> If you have not been sued yet, do your best to get the *Consent to Settle* clause in your policy.

It increases your malpractice premiums. Too many settlements can even make it difficult for you to be employed in the future.

Technically, your insurance company is not working for you but for themselves, to limit the risk of a large verdict. If they think a low settlement will save them money in the long run, they will do so, sometimes irrespective of whether or not you have "a good case."

Therefore, if you do not have the right to refuse a settlement, you are at the whim of your insurance company (or possibly your employers if they purchased your policy for you).

If you do have this very important right, you may request to go to trial regardless of the insurance company wishes. After all, it is not their record that will be affected by a settlement. It is yours and yours alone. (For more on settlement, see Chapter 8, *Should you settle?*)

If you have not yet been sued and do not have this *Consent to Settle* clause in your policy at the present time, you should strive to get it in there if possible. Sometimes you do not have a choice, but it does not hurt to ask.

What are the options if your employer purchases your insurance policy and dictates the terms?

If you work for a company that has purchased a policy for you, or if you work for a company that is self-insured, then you likely have no say over what clauses go into your policy. If this is your situation, you have three options:

1 *Find out how aggressive they are in refusing to settle cases.* Many employers have realized that plaintiff's attorneys are less likely to take a case against physicians if they know that their employers have a reputation for taking every case to trial. If your company fights most of its lawsuits to the bitter end, you can feel a little better about not having that clause in your medical malpractice insurance policy.

2 *Purchase your own policy.* Some employers will adjust your salary upward if you refuse their malpractice coverage and instead purchase your own. However, most will not. You could purchase your own policy despite also being covered by your employer. Although most doctors may think this an insane financial decision—to turn down free medical malpractice coverage—some doctors do this knowing that the ability to make important decisions for themselves can outweigh the cut in income.

The decision becomes all the more important if your employer and codefendant is a hospital. In Chapter 3, I explain at length the dangers of having a hospital as your codefendant. The problem is compounded if they also control your policy and your decision-making ability.

There are risks to purchasing your own policy, as you are a grouping of one and may have higher rates than if you had others pooled with you. Or, a lawsuit could get your individual coverage severely limited or dropped altogether. However, if you have your own policy, you can control what terms are in it, and your employer will not have any say in your lawsuit decisions.

3 *Do not work for that company.* It is a hard decision, but sometimes it is best to not work for an employer that purchases your policy for you. If you are looking for a job, conventional wisdom typically states that if you can get someone else to pay for your medical malpractice policy, do so. I offer an alternative view: If you can purchase your own policy with terms that are acceptable, but get group rating through your employer and a higher salary to compensate, that is the best scenario.

SECOND: Call your insurance company to report the claim

By reporting a claim, you initiate the process of having the insurance company cover your legal expenses and any verdict against you. Although it is possible that the insurance company already knows about your claim from your employer, you still need to make the call yourself.

> Reporting the claim to the insurance company is the critical first step in a very long process.

There may have been some circumstances that led you to report the potential lawsuit to them months ago, and a file has already been created on this case. For instance, the plaintiff attorney might have sent a letter to you or to the hospital to demand money for a bad outcome. You may have found out that other physicians you know have received letters requesting medical records regarding a patient. Or, the plaintiff's attorney may have requested a copy of your chart. In all of these circumstances, your first step would be to call the insurance company. However, if you are asked to provide records, do not send them anything, initially, until you have had a chance to seek advice from your insurance company. They may assign you an attorney or they may tell you to make an exact copy of each and every page of your chart. If applicable, do not exclude memos or billing. Do not include correspondence regarding insurance and legal issues. You might need to be assigned counsel to decide how to handle what will likely become a lawsuit, and that process begins with calling your insurance company.

Also, if you have a claims-made insurance policy, reporting a possible future lawsuit would be a very smart thing to do. A claims-made policy means that you are covered only for claims that arise during the policy period, for example, while you are working for a specific employer. If a lawsuit should arise after the policy period, then you are not covered. Therefore, if a potential case is reported before an actual lawsuit, it will still count under your claims-made policy, even if you leave your job and the lawsuit is filed after your coverage ends.

The other type of policy, called an occurrence policy, means that the claim could be made years after the policy ends and still be covered because the occurrence was during the policy period. And therefore, for an occurrence policy the timing of reporting potential claims is less critical.

You can also call your employer out of courtesy, but resist the passive tactic of letting your employer take over the process for you. You should be dealing with the insurance company directly. As some physicians' policies are purchased on their behalf by their employer, there is the temptation for the employers to want to control everything.

However, it is still your policy, and you should not let your employer take over, even if they offer. Keep in mind, there may be a conflict of interest between you and your employer, especially if they are also a codefendant with you on the case. (For more about conflict of interest, see Chapter 3, *What is a conflict of interest and how do I resolve one?*)

This is your case and your career. Be proactive. If your employer is a codefendant, do not allow them to act as an intermediary with the insurance company.

The only one looking out for you is you.

An exception to the above-mentioned advice is that you may already have an attorney that you trust to represent you. In that case, it is acceptable to have your attorney contact the insurance company for you to initiate the claim.

When you speak to the agents of your insurance company, they will likely ask you some details about the patient encounter if you have any specific recollections. The agents will ask you whether you believe any of the allegations are true. They will also likely ask if there are any other parties that have been sued along with you. Therefore, you should have read through the complaint to familiarize yourself with it and get an idea of why you are being sued. However, it is possible, if not likely, that after reading the complaint, you still may not know why you have been sued. Do not worry about that; there is plenty of time to do research that will help your recall. It is okay that you do not have your defense planned yet.

A few things to avoid

Do not look anything up in a book, journal, or an online site

You cannot give into this understandable temptation to find information that will help you justify your actions relative to whatever complaint is made against you.

You may think finding data to support your case will help bolster your confidence, as it is likely at an all time low, but it can be damaging to your case.

Here is why: When you are deposed (when a witness has sworn testimony taken outside of a courtroom without a judge present), and also at trial, the plaintiff's attorney will try to pin you down to an *authoritative source* of information. In other words, they will ask you, "Do you consider e.g. *Tintanelli* on Emergency Medicine, or *Harrison's* on Internal Medicine, authoritative texts?" Plaintiff's counsel might ask you what texts of your field are in your office or in your home.

Once you have disclosed that you have an authoritative source, the plaintiff's attorney at trial will embarrass you on the stand with obscure and out of context quotes that hurt your case.

Prevent this occurrence by saying this mantra over and over, *Nothing is authoritative.*

Books are out of date when printed. Journals are not gospel, not even if it is the *New England Journal of Medicine*. Reputable journals in other fields are not always relevant. Articles in journals are often flawed studies. Information is changing all the time.

There is a time to look up information: after meeting with your attorney. After consulting with your legal counsel, any research you do is for them, not you, and not subject to discovery (this may vary by state, and therefore, you should ask your attorney to be sure).

The plaintiff's attorney will try, at your deposition, to pin you down to an authoritative source. When you have deflected that issue, they will then ask you if you researched anything about the case after receiving the complaint. You will say, "No. I only looked up information per the request of my attorney." Your attorney (if any good) will then object to any attempts to find out any more information on this topic. You will then have frustrated the plaintiff and helped your case a great deal, a two for one special.

Other advice: (1) do not talk to anyone other than your attorney or your spouse about the details of your case and (2) do not destroy or alter evidence.

Do not talk to anyone

You can talk to your attorney and your spouse about the specifics of the case. However, anyone else you speak to about this case can be called or deposed as witnesses.

Specifically, do not speak to your colleagues about this case unless it is in a peer-review setting. Anything you say to them outside of peer review is not protected and can certainly be used against you. (See Chapter 15 for more information on peer review.)

You might think about talking to that surgeon who found the appendicitis you missed. Don't. No matter what they may say to you that seems supportive of your care, you never really know if they will be helpful to you. It is best to keep that door closed, because once opened, it can hurt your case significantly.

Also, do not contact the plaintiff or their attorney. You may think you have "proof" that can convince them to drop your case. And you might. However, it is a risky tactic that could set up a situation where the case continues and your proof of innocence is now not admissible. If you have any evidence you think could get your case dropped, show it to your attorney and let them figure out the best method of using it.

An example: Doctor X always makes sure to tape-record all conversations with his patients involving informed consent (with full disclosure to the patient that the taping is occurring). At a later date, the physician is sued by a patient claiming that he did not explain the procedure he was going to do and that her negative outcome was completely unexpected. The physician's tape is the kind of proof that can get a case dismissed.

Also, your attorney is now your official representative in all matters regarding this case. You are not to talk with the plaintiff outside of an organized legal setting. The time for apologies has passed. (For more about apologies, see Chapter 11, *If something goes wrong, should I apologize?*)

Although you may think that a conversation between the two of you, without your attorneys, could change their mind and get them to drop the case, the true likelihood is infinitesimally small. The only thing it will accomplish is getting your actions and words twisted around to make you look very bad in your deposition and in court.

Do not destroy or alter evidence

You may think that cleverly adding some information to the chart may help you. However, in all likelihood, a copy of the original exists somewhere you do not even realize, and it will resurface during trial to annihilate you.

If you have additional documentation, such as a personal diary, that you think could hurt your case, now is not the time to destroy it. Although it is a bad idea to keep a diary (this is explained further in Chapter 13), once you are sued, it is too late. You may think no one can discover that you destroyed evidence; however, clever attorneys will find out.

You never want to appear deceitful. If proof of your altering the chart or making other information disappear comes to light, your case is lost. Do not risk this. You would be surprised at how many physicians break this rule and lose big. Or settle big. For cases that were winnable.

Avoid the blame game

Do not blame yourself. I know it is not possible to go through the process of a lawsuit emotionally unscathed; however, you must try your best to realize that most physicians get sued at some point in their career. Often, more than once. Just because you have been sued, it does not mean you are a bad doctor.

Do not blame your patients. The worst possible sequela of a medical malpractice lawsuit is the destruction of the trust between doctor and patient.

> It is a natural reaction to want to assign blame: to yourself, your patients, or the "evil" plaintiff's attorneys.

It will be difficult to put this case aside, but do your best not to look at your patients as "the enemy."

Do not lose your compassion. It is easy to let the painful process of a lawsuit take over your emotions and make you bitter.

Try to remember why you went into medicine in the first place: to help people. Compassionate doctors, in my opinion, are the best doctors. Bitter doctors, who do not care about their patients, make bad doctors. (They also get poor patient satisfaction numbers and more angry patients that can lead to future lawsuits; see Chapter 11.)

Do your best to retain (or regain) your compassion despite all the obstacles thrown your way. It will keep you sane and make you a better doctor. Do not forget you are the same compassionate competent physician today as you were yesterday.

Do not change your quality practice of medicine. There are many courses out there for physicians that give recommendations to avoid lawsuits. Unfortunately, sometimes the "defensible" way to treat a patient is not necessarily the best medical practice.

Try to avoid following medicolegal advice that goes against the good medical treatment that you provide to your patients just because an "expert" in a course said so.

For instance, a colleague once told me that they would not take a signout from me because they do not do incision and drainage (I&D) on the face.

When a person has an abscess, it is the recommended practice to perform an I&D. If not performed, the abscess might not resolve despite antibiotic administration.

My colleague's refusal was based on a medicolegal course where the instructor said never to do I&Ds on the face because of the possibility of causing a scar on the face that would lead to a lawsuit. Never mind that an inappropriately treated abscess would eventually lead to a bigger scar! I found this appalling, both that the advice was given *and* that the advice was taken.

In matters of medicine, I understand that there are many instances where the most defensible means of treatment is not necessarily the best medical practice. But we took an oath, and I believe that following best practice *is* the best and most defensible in the long run. The best methodology is when good medical practice is also defensible medical practice.

If a patient insists on a test that you do not feel they need, in particular computed tomography (CT) scans, it may not be wise medicolegally to refuse. However, it is always prudent to explain the radiation risks involved in CT scanning: that a small but significant number of patients undergoing a CT scan will develop cancer from the CT scan. (Make sure to document that you explained the risks of a CT scan.)

Getting sued can damage your self-confidence. However, do not let fear consume you. Make every effort to continue practicing the good medicine you have been doing for years.

It is possible that the lawsuit is a result of your unintentional negligence. If that is the case, realize you are human. We all make mistakes. It may feel unfair that physicians can be sued for those errors when there are scores of people (e.g., politicians) who make errors in judgment daily, which cause irreversible harm to people, yet are exempt from such lawsuits. But, unfortunately, this is our reality.

Sometimes, you need to be introspective and decide if something about the way you practice medicine needs to be altered to give better treatment to patients. Sometimes, there is nothing that can be done.

Sometimes nothing *should* be done, as your "error" was really a statistical reality and you are already practicing the best medicine possible.

Statistically every doctor will experience bad outcomes. And because physicians are human, they will make errors. You are not alone.

Therefore, what is the difference between a predictable bad outcome and a medical malpractice? See Chapter 2 for more information.

Chapter 2 **What is medical malpractice?**

The term *medical malpractice* can mean different things to different people. The American Medical Association defines it as "a doctor's failure to exercise the degree of care and skill that a physician and surgeon of the same medical specialty would use under similar circumstances" (http://virtualmentor. ama-assn.org/2007/06/hlaw1-0706.html). Patients often confuse a bad outcome with negligent care on the part of the physician. Combine bad luck and an inaccessible physician with a condescending attitude, and a lawsuit is sure to follow.

> A bad outcome does not mean you committed negligence, even though this may be why you were sued.

Physicians (especially those who have been sued) view most errors as an expected statistical reality. Many are systemic problems rather than doctor-specific problems. Some are simply bad luck. As human beings, we are not expected to be perfect. However, there are some situations that even a physician would agree with as being malpractice.

An example of medical malpractice is when physicians insist on treating a condition that is not in their specialty and thus cause damage. Another obvious circumstance of medical malpractice is when the physician is impaired by drugs or alcohol but still continues to treat patients. Performing unnecessary procedures just to make money is another unmistakable example of malpractice.

The plaintiff's attorneys justify their practice as a way to police the medical system and weed out bad doctors. However, based on the statistics, this is not what is happening. According to the National Practitioner Data Bank (NPDB), during the time period September 1, 1990, through September 30, 2002,

How to Survive a Medical Malpractice Lawsuit. By © Ilene R. Brenner. Published 2010 Blackwell Publishing.

only 5% of doctors were responsible for 54% of malpractice payouts. Yet during that same time period the NPDB found that only 8% of doctors with two or more malpractice payouts had been disciplined by their state medical board, and only 17% of doctors with *five* or more malpractice payouts had been disciplined by their state medical board.

> Only a very small percentage of physicians commit "legally defined" malpractice.

Clearly, there are different opinions on what is considered medical malpractice. However, the law has clear guidelines as to what is required to win a case against a physician. If these are met, the physicians are said to be liable for their actions.

There are four criteria that make up a successful claim against a physician: duty, breach, proximate cause, and damages. (Some states such as New York have only three criteria: liability, proximate cause, and damages.)

Duty

The physician must have an obligation to treat that patient. One instance where a physician might not have a duty to treat a particular patient is during the "drive-by consult." In other words, when physicians not on call are asked their opinion by the emergency physician, there is no legal contract that binds them to that patient. Physicians on the hospital call list do have a duty to treat patients presenting to the emergency department even if they have never seen the patient previously.

Once physician–patient relationship has been established, physicians have the duty to possess and apply the medical knowledge and skills required of a reasonably competent medical practitioner engaged in the same specialty. In addition, physicians must show that they use medical judgment in the exercise of their care as would be consistent with that of a reasonably competent practitioner in the same specialty. This is what is commonly referred to as following the *standard of care*.

If physicians want to discharge a patient from their practice, they must make reasonable arrangements for continuation of the patient's care by another physician or else it could be construed as abandonment of their duty.

> Patients can terminate their relationship with the doctor at any time for any reason. Physicians must give specific reasons for releasing a patient from their care after providing formal notice and giving the patient a reasonable time period to find another physician.

Other examples of patient abandonment are as follows: (A) failing to transfer a patient who needs specialty care you cannot provide to the proper physician/facility and (B) failing to respond to phone calls from nurses in the hospital who are taking care of your patient.

Breach

In this case, your care was not in accordance with the good and acceptable medical practice for your specialty. Another way of expressing this concept is as a *breach of duty*. This is perhaps the most subjective of the criteria as the standard of care is not always clear. In medicine, there are certain facts and treatments that are universally accepted. However, medical practice evolves and changes frequently based on new evidence. Different specialties can treat the same diagnosis in different ways based on their own biases.

In addition, clinical judgment calls, though found in retrospect to be in error, will usually not be considered a deviation from the standard of care provided the physician used their best medical knowledge or judgment. Communicating this subtle fact to a jury is one of the most challenging aspects of a trial.

The way the courts determine standard of care is through expert testimony. Again, "expert" is a nebulous term as each state has different guidelines for defining an expert (see Appendix A). For instance, an internist should not be able to give expert testimony on a neurosurgical case. However, in many states this is allowed. For more information on experts, see Chapter 4.

Proximate cause

This definition varies between states in a subtle but important way: (A) your care had to be *the* cause of the patient's injury or (B) your care had to be *a* cause of the patient's injury. How you define it clearly makes it easier or harder to prove the proximate cause criteria of a medical malpractice lawsuit. For instance, if your care had to be *the* cause of the patient's injury, then it means that if there are other causes of the injury, your negligent care would not be the only reason for the injury and thus proximate cause could not be claimed against you. But if the definition is broadened to *a* cause, and if your negligence had any part in causing that injury, then the proximate cause criteria can be sustained against you.

> Proximate cause is defined legally as a causative element which, in a natural and continuous sequence, unbroken by any intervening event, produces injury, and without which, the injury would not have occurred.

There are many situations where a physician could be liable for negligent care, but the physician's care did not cause the injury. In a real-life example, an internist had an X-ray taken on a patient who presented with a cough. It was read as negative, but it was actually abnormal. One year later, the patient died from adenocarcinoma of the lung. In this situation, it was shown that as of the date of X-ray, the adenocarcinoma was already metastasized, and no form of treatment would have affected the outcome. Therefore, even though the physician missed the diagnosis of cancer, there is no proximate cause. The patient was already beyond the point of being helped when presented to the doctor, so there was nothing that was going to change the course of this patient's prognosis.

In reality, cases that are defended solely on the basis of lack of proximate cause are very hard to win. Although the law may be in your favor, it is hard to convince a jury that though the doctor misdiagnosed the patient, and the patient died, there is actually no medical malpractice.

Damages

The issue of damages is a little bit more straightforward. In this case, there must be a compensable injury (i.e., involving monetary damages). There are two types of damages: economic and noneconomic. Economic damages are monetary issues such as lost wages or hospital bills. Noneconomic damages include subjective issues such as pain and suffering.

> Although rare, medical malpractice cases can involve punitive damages. These are awarded only to inflict an economic punishment on defendants who the jury feels have acted recklessly or maliciously.

There are many instances where no damages occur even though there was breach of duty and proximate cause. An example would be the physician who prescribed the wrong medicine dosage, which the patient took, but no harm occurred.

In another instance, if you have a nursing home patient who has severe dementia and is contracted and immobile from an old stroke, and a subsequent treating physician failed to diagnose a new stroke, but the patient's status remained the same, there would be no damages.

Conversely, you can have a case where there are severe damages but no liability. These situations tend to occur most often with brain-damaged babies. Many times a baby suffers a brain injury, and it is not the fault of the physician. These are very emotional cases, which, if lost, go for millions of dollars.

In an actual lawsuit, a pregnant patient was told by her physician to come to hospital at the first sign of any pains. However, the patient did not come to hospital in a timely manner because she was waiting for a babysitter for her other children. When she finally reached the hospital and delivered, the cord was prolapsed (the complication in which the umbilical cord falls into the birth canal ahead of the baby's head or other parts of the baby's body and gets compressed), which caused hypoxia. This led to the baby's subsequent brain damage. Whatever the physician attempted to do, there was nothing that could have prevented this bad outcome. It was the delay in seeking care that led to baby's brain damage. So there was no breach of duty or proximate cause, though huge potential damages.

Minimizing the potential for liability is the cornerstone of lawsuit prevention. The examples of situations for which a physician has increased liability are numerous and are addressed in much more detail in Section 2 "An Ounce of Prevention." However, I will give a few notable examples in the following text.

The first example addresses phone consults. Are you liable for giving advice to another physician on the phone for a patient you have never seen? If you are on call when you are paged, it is your duty to give advice, and therefore, you can share in liability for an adverse outcome that results from your advice. However, if you are not on call, and are then asked for advice, you have no duty toward the patient, and your liability is much more limited.

In another example, if a patient was assigned to your service as an inpatient, but never shows up in your office for the scheduled appointments, will you be liable for any worsening of the patient's condition? Unfortunately, the answer is yes. You may be liable because it is the same illness that you treated in the hospital, and therefore, you still have a duty to treat this patient, and anything bad that happens could be interpreted as a breach of duty.

A suggestion to minimize this liability is that if you are the doctor whose patient has two missed appointments postdischarge from the hospital, you must send a certified letter that states, "You have missed your last two appointments that my office scheduled for you. Your condition is potentially serious and could worsen if not monitored. If you do not reschedule and see me in my office soon, I cannot be responsible for what will likely be further deterioration of your condition." However, despite this letter, you must follow up with phone calls and then document in the patient's chart that these phone calls happened. If you are ever sued, you can subpoena your office phone records to prove that these calls were made.

Finally, in-office X-rays offer huge potentials for liability. Many orthopedists and internists have bought or leased X-ray machines and saved the patient from having to go to the hospital for this simple procedure. However, while the process of taking an X-ray may be relatively simple, the reading process may not be. Physicians who read their own X-rays obviously feel qualified to read them without any radiologist oversight. But are they?

Certainly most orthopedists would say that for what they do, they read the X-rays as good or better than the radiologist. And that may be true. However, would most internists suggest that they feel qualified to see a small dot on the chest X-ray and differentiate this as a normal marking versus early cancer? As it is, many radiologists miss subtle findings such as this. Is an internist trained well enough in X-ray reading to make this distinction? This is certainly a subject for debate. What is not debatable is the fact that many internists are sued for missing lung cancer in its earliest stages.

Therefore, having in-office X-ray machines does increase your liability, and you need to weigh the value of having this technology available to your patients versus the increased risk of being sued. To lessen the liability, you could decide to have radiology overreads for X-rays performed in your office. However, having a radiologist *officially* read your X-rays after a day or two might not be financially viable for a small-office practice as insurers will not pay for your X-ray reading if a radiologist reads it as well.

Are EMTALA issues considered medical malpractice?

EMTALA is an acronym that stands for The Emergency Medical Treatment and Active Labor Act. The statute was enacted by congress to prevent patient dumping and discrimination against uninsured patients by hospitals. Before EMTALA, it was a regular occurrence for hospitals to turn away sick uninsured patients. Triage consisted of a *wallet biopsy* (finding out if the patient is insured), and if a male, then the first question on history asked was about military service, which would require transfer to the Veterans Affairs (VA) hospital.

EMTALA requires that a medical screening exam should be conducted before turning away the patient from the hospital, and it also governs transfers from one hospital to another. A hospital that participates in Medicare and is found to violate EMTALA can be fined and could possibly face termination of its Medicare provider agreement. Physician penalties for violating EMTALA are variable.

Physicians could be fined or subject their hospital to fines if found to violate EMTALA, as well as face exclusion from Medicare and Medicaid. However, physicians can also be subject to a civil lawsuit for negligence under the personal injury guidelines in the state where the violation occurred.

EMTALA has many implications for malpractice claims. It does not take the place or limit a malpractice claim under state law. Although the facts that led to an EMTALA violation could be used to file a civil claim against the physician, the EMTALA violation itself is not the ground for a lawsuit. It is, however, admissible at trial and could be very influential to a jury.

EMTALA creates an opportunity for the plaintiff to have a second avenue for which to make a claim for damages. Also, the plaintiff can use EMTALA to get the claim heard in federal court. (There is more on the difference between federal and state courts later on in this chapter and in Chapter 5.) Although various rulings are not clear, it does not appear that tort reform limits on noneconomic damages apply in EMTALA cases. (A tort is a legal wrong; negligence and medical malpractice lawsuits are in the tort area. Thus, tort reform is a legal means to discourage the filing of lawsuits by making plaintiff's attorneys be more selective in the cases they take.) As EMTALA cases are usually not affected by tort reform pain and suffering monetary limits, the plaintiff has an added incentive to file an EMTALA claim in addition to the medical malpractice claim in states where such limits exist.

What about a complaint to the medical board? Is that considered malpractice?

A lawsuit is not the only way that a patient can use to express dissatisfaction with your care. Although infrequent, patients can make complaints to the medical licensing board in your state.

The prospect of a lawsuit may be a terrifying experience; however, a complaint that could directly affect your license is worse. Although anyone can make a complaint, typically complaints are made by patients or their family members. This can happen outside of a lawsuit, or it could be after a physician settlement or loss. What kinds of complaints will a board review? This depends on the state, but as a general rule they will evaluate unprofessional behavior, patient endangerment, and working while under the influence of alcohol or drugs.

> Although rudeness to patients may be unprofessional, most medical boards do not consider it a punishable offense.

In addition, the board can investigate you without an actual complaint. Many states have a system in place that flags physicians in the event that there was a settlement or loss for a large amount of money or if a physician were to have multiple settlements or losses within a short period of time (e.g., five settlements in 3 years). You will likely receive a letter from the board detailing the nature of the complaint against you. Depending on your state, you may be able to resolve the complaint with an acceptable written explanation.

If not, you will have a hearing in front of the state medical board. There is no judge. There is no jury. You can have an attorney to represent you. Your medical malpractice insurance coverage typically covers the costs for representation. Although there can be fines, there is no compensation given to the patient making the complaint.

Usually the board is made up of physicians from various fields. Does this mean that a urologist who is brought before the board will have a urologist on the panel? Not necessarily. Does this seem unfair? It may appear that way, but actually, it may be to your benefit *not* to have a physician in your field on the panel.

Although this may seem counterintuitive, there is some logic to this. As a general rule, a physician in your field will be more critical of your behavior. They know much more about the specific facts involved in your complaint and tend to judge much more harshly as a result. However, that knowledge of the minutia may taint the bigger issues in your case. Also, they will have added influence on the other members of the board who may not have as clear knowledge of your specialty. Probably, your complaint will be dismissed. If not, there are many possibilities for disciplinary action. Suspension or revocation of physician license is the most severe, of course. More minor actions could include corrective procedures, fines, and probation.

Is there an alternative way to resolve a lawsuit?

As a result of the current medical liability crisis of skyrocketing premiums and limited access to insurance, various tort reform measures were enacted in states across the United States. Many of those solutions included alternative dispute resolution (ADR) methods through which a complaint can be resolved without litigation. The various techniques range from voluntary to mandated choices, binding to nonbinding outcomes, and from processes that are less likely to disrupt personal and professional life to those that are more public and intrusive. There are a number of risks and benefits associated with the four main ADR processes (see Appendix B for a listing of states that have ADR laws in place).

Various types of ADRs:
- negotiation
- mediation
- arbitration
- pretrial screening panel

Negotiation

This is the most frequently used ADR and is defined as the process whereby two or more parties confer together in good faith so as to settle a matter of mutual concern. One of the major advantages of negotiation is that those resolutions tend to have greater durability than agreements reached by other methods. Also, those involved have a much greater control of the process. Negotiation tends to be more successful when those involved are agents of those involved and thus have sufficient emotional distance to compromise. However, in medical malpractice cases, it can be difficult to get the dispassionate perspective that is conducive to successful resolution through negotiation alone.

Mediation

Mediation is an extension of direct negotiation between the parties, using a neutral third party to facilitate the negotiation process. The mediator has no authority to impose a solution on the parties, nor are the results of the process binding, as they are simply a facilitator of the negotiation. This method can be effective in medical malpractice cases in which the patient and physician want to preserve their relationship or in which poor communication has led to the dispute. There are many advantages of mediation over litigation, which include decreased costs, more control over the process by the disputing parties, and more confidential proceedings. Patients tend to favor mediation as a forum in which they can express their concerns and may lead to an acknowledgement of the problem—oftentimes with just a simple apology. On the contrary, there are limitations such as its voluntary nature, lack of a judge that can impose the decisions, and the fact that a mediator has only as much power as the disputing parties permit.

Arbitration

This form of resolution occurs when the parties agree to submit their dispute to an arbitration panel or an arbitrator who conducts a hearing whereby each side presents evidence and a determination is made on liability and/or renders a decision of an award. Arbitration can be binding, but sometimes it is possible to appeal the result. It can be a private contract or judicially mandated. The process is usually faster, less costly, and more private than a jury trial. Also, a skilled arbitrator can be very knowledgeable in the complex medical terminology, which can make sorting through the dispute a fairer process than having a jury of laypersons who do not truly understand the issues involved. On the other hand, since as physicians win over 80% of the lawsuits that go to trial, the lack of jury involvement might not be to the physicians' advantage.

Pretrial screening panel

This resolution method was developed specifically for medical malpractice cases. A large number of states have statutes establishing pretrial screening panels that review medical malpractice claims and render a nonbinding advisory opinion on the merits of the claim before a suit is filed. Panel composition varies considerably by state and can consist of only physicians, only attorneys, or a combination of both with a possibility of judges and laypersons participating as well. Also, a few states use the panel's decision as the expert testimony at trial (see Appendix B for more information). Its purpose is to eliminate nonmeritorious claims and to encourage settlement of legitimate claims before litigation. However, as the process is nonbinding, the plaintiff can still litigate after the decision is made, thus actually delay the final resolution of the claim.

> Although many states have avenues for various types of ADR, understand that any payments that are made will be reported to the NPDB. This is a major barrier to the widespread acceptance of ADR.

Every time a physician seeks or renews privileges at a hospital, the NPDB may be queried and it could harm your job prospects. These settlements could affect your liability insurance by raising your rates or limiting your practice. Plus, it could trigger a review by your state medical board. Most physicians would rather play the high odds of winning at trial over the riskier proposition of submitting to ADR (Fraser and the Committee on Medical Liability, 2001).

Regardless of how a patient makes a complaint against you, whether through the legal system or through the medical board, or resolves the dispute through ADR, it is imperative you have a good attorney to defend you. Chapter 3 details how to choose the right attorney for you, and how to get a new attorney if you do not like the one you were assigned.

Reference

Fraser JJ Jr, the Committee on Medical Liability. American Academy of Pediatrics: Technical report: Alternative dispute resolution in medical malpractice. Pediatrics 2001;107(3):602–7.

Chapter 3 **How to choose an attorney**

You have been sued and are working your way through the various avenues of the legal process. Now you have to evaluate your representation. How do you know if you have the right attorney? This is a tough question because it is like asking for a recommendation for a good doctor; it is pretty subjective. But there are a few questions you can ask your prospective attorney that will make your choice clearer.

Q1. Are you a partner?

Senior partners are ideal, but any partner should be adequate. The logic is that defense trial attorneys typically make partners based on a history of winning the majority of their cases. Unless the person has a family connection with the firm's owner, a defense trial attorney had to earn the partnership.

Q2. What is your win/loss ratio?

The reasoning for this is obvious. However, there is a caveat where some lawyers have great ratios because they try lower level cases. Some lawyers have unfavorable ratios because they try the most difficult cases.

Q3. Have you tried any cases similar to mine?

The more times they have handled your type of case, the better they will try yours. However, a good attorney can always learn the medicine; therefore, it is not necessarily a deal breaker if they have not tried a case similar to yours.

How to Survive a Medical Malpractice Lawsuit. By © Ilene R. Brenner. Published 2010 Blackwell Publishing.

> You want trial-experienced attorneys, preferably partners, who represent
> doctors rather than hospitals most of the time.

Q4. Do most of your cases entail representing hospitals?

If so, this is not the firm for you. Hospitals often settle out of the case early;
therefore, if attorneys handle that type of situation as their main "trial
experience," they will likely have problems trying a case from a doctor's
perspective.

In addition, hospitals are often sued as the location of the malpractice
that happens to have deep pockets. They are not often targeted as the sole
cause of medical malpractice. Therefore, attorneys who represent mostly hospitals will not be properly battle tested with all the pressures and stresses of a
"target" doctor.

When attorneys represent hospitals, they are representing a faceless organization without anything more than money at risk. Representing physicians
is much more personal and has more serious considerations such as future
ability to obtain insurance and retaining medical licensure. Attorneys who
represent hospitals may not be much sensitive to the emotional aspects of a
lawsuit.

In addition, there are many psychological conflicts that go on before and
during the trial and you want an attorney who is used to these games and who
plays to win.

Q5. Over the last 5 years, have you settled a majority of your cases?

Again, this goes to trial experience. You could have lawyers with many years
post–law school, but if they are not trying many cases and not having experience, in all likelihood, they will not be very good.

A large number of cases in medical malpractice situations go to trial and
verdict. If your attorney has settled most of the cases handled, then it is
likely that he or she is trying lower level cases and may be learning the trade.
This type of attorney may pressure you to settle marginal but defensible
cases rather than go to verdict for fear of losing and looking bad.

Q6. Have you tried any cases in federal court?

This is relevant only if your case was filed in federal court instead of the
more common situation of the lawsuit being in state court. There are many
differences, some subtle and many drastically different (see Chapter 8 for a

discussion of the differences between federal court and state court). You do not want your attorney learning the specifics of federal civil procedure on the fly during your case.

As a general rule, you want an older, experienced trial attorney who typically represents doctors. It is important that you understand that first-time defendant physicians will likely have a law firm assigned to them by the insurance company. However, the above-mentioned questions can help you decide if the attorney assigned to your case is adequate. For instance, if you are given a low-level attorney with little trial experience, you can insist on a partner.

If you have thoroughly evaluated your assigned law firm and wish to change, follow the strategies listed in the next section. However, I would like to point out that your insurance company has an interest in a successful outcome for your case. Therefore, it is likely that any law firm listed on their panel is competent. However, sometimes, one firm is a better fit for you than the other.

> If there is even a whiff of conflict of interest, you must insist on your own attorney.

What is a conflict of interest and how do I resolve one?

Let us assume that you found a "good attorney." You still may not want to use him or her. Particularly, if he or she was assigned to you by the insurance company.

For instance, if you are not the only defendant in the case, multiple-defendant situations complicate matters tremendously. Often, insurance companies will assign the same attorney to all the codefendants in the case. From their perspective, it saves money for them as there is less duplication of efforts (and hours billed).

However, if you think that your codefendants may bear some fault, you may need your own representation separate from them. This is especially important if your codefendants happen to be partners of yours or are partners in your employer's company.

Although lawyers are supposed to be fair to all parties, if your company gives them a considerable degree of business, your lawyer may not pursue a defense tactic for you that your bosses do not like.

Take for example that there are three defendants, doctor 1, doctor 2, and doctor corporate entity (this can include the hospital), and assume there are multiple defense tactics available—(a) favorable to doctor 1, (b) favorable to doctor 2, (c) favorable to corporation, and (d) equal favorability to all. If one attorney is assigned to all defendants, then the most likely defense tactic will be "d" (also "c" if the corporation gives the attorney a considerable degree of business, as mentioned earlier). However, if each entity had its own attorney, and if you were doctor 1, then you would get a defense tactic most closely tailored to your specific needs (scenario "a").

The more defendants in your case, the higher the likelihood of a conflict of interest.

Obviously, it is still necessary to work with one another as defendants to provide a united front. But in the end, as I said earlier, the only one looking out for you is you. There may come a time in the case where your best chance at a defendant's verdict is at the detriment of one of your codefendants.

However, in the majority of situations, it is not a problem to have multiple doctors represented by one attorney. One advantage of having all parties represented by the same attorney is that all the defendants will be "on the same page."

What I mean by this: Part of the reason a plaintiff's attorney sues multiple entities is to increase the chance that someone will be found to be at fault. Also, it creates deep pockets of insurance coverage. Thus, it is to the plaintiff's advantage to have the defendants attack one another. With one attorney representing all parties, it is unlikely the finger-pointing will take place.

Although you may weigh the pros and cons of seeking separate counsel with doctor and corporate codefendants, there is one situation where YOU SHOULD GET YOUR OWN SEPARATE COUNSEL: IF YOUR HOSPITAL IS A CODEFENDANT.

Under this circumstance, if you have the opportunity to get your own representation at another law firm, do so! Your hospital codefendant can screw you in so many ways, it is not even funny! Here's how.

Your hospital codefendant can be your worst enemy:
- magic witnesses
- putting your job in jeopardy
- pressure to settle
- indemnification

Magic witnesses

Witnesses, which were never mentioned before, magically materialize at trial to point the finger at you. They have perfect memories but no documentation to back it up. This happens all the time. This will happen whether you have the same attorney or not. But if you have your own attorney, he or she can at least anticipate this and defend you. If you have the same attorney, they'll dump on you (in other words, key witnesses for the defense will say things that implicate you rather than your codefendants), and you will not have any way to protect yourself.

Putting your job in jeopardy

Your hospital can try to threaten your job if you choose a particular defense. Some attorneys might not consider that defense if representing both of you (see the scenarios mentioned earlier). Better to lose your job than lose your case. You can always get another job. But once you are in the data bank, you are there forever.

In a similar vein, if you have the same attorney, the hospital may *choose* your defense for you. The attorney will take care of the "big gun," the hospital, and you will be hung out to dry.

Pressure to settle

The hospital could put pressure on you to settle. Even if you are an employee of the hospital, you need not have to settle just because the hospital does. They often do it for monetary reasons. But if you have a reasonably good case, it is better to press on to verdict. Remember, a settlement is a loss for the doctor. (For more on settlement, see Chapter 8, *Should You settle?*)

Indemnification

If you were a hospital employee, then the hospital may sue you if you lose the case. This is called indemnification. Here is how it works: Assume you have a $1,000,000 policy. If the jury comes in and finds the doctor 50% liable and the hospital 50% liable, then they are both jointly liable and each has to be responsible for this verdict (if you live in a state that assigns joint and several liability). Therefore, in a $10,000,000 verdict, the doctor's $1,000,000 limit would be covered by his or her policy, and the other $4,000,000 would be covered by the hospital's policy. The hospital actually pays 9 million dollars of the 10 million dollar verdict.

Because the payouts are not 50/50 despite the equal liability, the hospital now can (and sometimes will) sue you for the extra 4 million dollars that were not its share of the verdict. Do you have insurance to defend you against the hospital? Not likely.

It should be understood that the hospital has bigger pockets. It will shoulder a larger percentage of the liability. As a result, it will be more inclined to settle a case, even if there is a good shot of winning.

Therefore, there is a likely conflict of interest between you and the hospital. It is for this reason that you should have private counsel.

How do I change my attorney?

If you have a situation where you are unhappy with your attorney, but the law firm is reputable, you may want to simply exchange attorneys within the same law firm. Before you get to the point of asking for a switch, you need to find out if the attorney handling the initial complaint is the same attorney that will be handling your deposition and trial.

Often, large firms assign junior attorneys the initial complaint. However, at the deposition and trial, you should have a more experienced attorney such as a partner or a senior associate who has significant trial skills. On your initial meeting with the attorneys, when you ask questions evaluating their appropriateness for your case, you should make it very clear that you expect senior, experienced trial attorneys to be conducting the deposition and trial.

It is possible that the attorneys will tell you that they are more than qualified to try your case and attempt to assuage your concerns. However, they should agree to switch to another attorney if you insist.

Defense-oriented medical malpractice law firms exist on doctors' referrals. Your law firm will look at you as both an existing client and a potential new referral in the future. Many small firms exist only on referrals from happy and satisfied clients, essentially someone like you. You are a current and future cash cow. They will or should accommodate you for that reason alone.

If they will not comply, find out who their supervising attorney is and contact them. Keep going up the chain of command until you either (1) get the experienced attorney you desired or (2) are given a complete run-around.

Any law firm that does not agree to give you a senior attorney when you request it *should* be dropped in favor of one that will. See the next section for specific instructions.

How do I change law firms?

If after reading the article this far you realize that you do not wish to keep this particular law firm, you need to find out what your options are. In

Chapter 1, I explained that you need to find out if your policy allows you to select your own law firm.

There are two possibilities:

• *First possibility*: Your policy might say that you CANNOT choose your attorney/law firm. This does not necessarily mean you are stuck.

Your first step is to call your insurance company representatives and ask them to switch law firms. If they do not agree, continue to go up the chain of command and demand, both verbally and in writing, your specific reasons for wanting to switch law firms.

When conversing with the insurance company representatives, use terms such as "conflict of interest" liberally. Once they hear that (and see it in writing, MAKE SURE YOU HAVE IT IN WRITING), they will often acquiesce. This will scare them into thinking that you will register a complaint against them to the state insurance department in the event you lose, on the grounds that there was a conflict of interest that they knew about and ignored. This alone is usually sufficient because, generally, insurance companies do not like unhappy doctors. Unfortunately, there are some insurance companies that will not concede despite your best efforts. At this point, you must play hardball with your assigned law firm.

You will then need to draft a letter to one of the senior partners that states your complaint and insists that they recuse themselves from your case. Be sure to state in your letter, "If you refuse to remove yourself from my case and I lose because of the conflict of interest, I will report you to the state bar association." Therefore, this final recourse should get them to drop you as a client.

• *Second possibility*: Your policy may say that you CAN choose your attorney/law firm. Or, it may not mention the topic at all. In this case, you should insist on another attorney. However, this is not always as easy as it sounds.

Summary of how to get your own attorney separate from your codefendants if you think there is a conflict of interest:
 – Ask the insurance company representative.
 – If they refuse, keep making noise with their superiors.
 – Use the term "conflict of interest" liberally.
 – Ask your attorney to recuse themselves if you still are not successful.
 – Put all your requests in writing.

Insurance companies may still try to bully you into thinking that what they say goes. Again, it is in their best interest to spend as little money as possible on the defense and they would rather have everyone represented by one lawyer. Do not accept their refusal.

In this situation, you can follow the above-mentioned steps *and* you can threaten the insurance company with a lawsuit for breach of contract. These may seem like extreme measures, but if that is what it takes to get adequate representation, it is a necessary maneuver.

In sum, you want a good, experienced trial attorney, preferably a partner, who represents doctors most of the time. And if there is even a whiff of a conflict of interest, you must insist on your own attorney.

It is imperative you feel secure in your representation. So much about the lawsuit is stressful. Having a confident, compassionate attorney looking out for your best interest will help alleviate many of the anxieties that you will experience. Chapter 4 goes into much more detail on the emotional toll of a lawsuit.

Chapter 4 **Coping with a medical malpractice lawsuit**

When faced with the prospect of a medical malpractice lawsuit, you will likely experience a multitude of emotions. And although the road in front of you seems long and dark, there are proven ways of coping. It is best to lay aside the hurt and anger that you understandably feel. Handle this as the attorneys do. Nothing is personal; it is just a game. One in which the client with the best attorney often wins.

Sure, it sounds easy, and yet it is very hard. People commonly quote statistics that upwards of 80% of all cases are won by the defendant (AMA website, medical liability reform fast facts http://www.ama-assn.org/ama1/pub/upload/mm/399/mlr_fastfacts.pdf—is actually referenced from Physician Insurers Association of America, 2005). But for us, the physician, the moment we get sued, we have already lost on some level; our compassion, our idealism, and our very self-confidence is at risk.

The physicians' most precious asset, time, fritters away because of many hours spent defending their case. As will be described in the course of this book, the physicians will spend many unreimbursed hours in discussions with their attorney for deposition and trial preparation. However, the physicians will spend many more hours outside of their attorney's office researching issues relevant to their case.

> There is a huge emotional toll that occurs from this long multiyear process.

For most physicians, once they have been sued, the lawsuit is never far from their thoughts. The periods of "quiet" where nothing happens with the case are simply the calm before the storm. Even free time away from the case is stolen away as you cannot help but run the case over and over in your mind considering the ramifications of a negative outcome.

How to Survive a Medical Malpractice Lawsuit. By © Ilene R. Brenner. Published 2010 Blackwell Publishing.

Understandably, there are worries about financial security and career viability. Obstetricians know that they are only one plaintiff's verdict away from enormous liability insurance premiums that obviate their future ability to deliver babies. Other physicians worry that they may not be able to join another group because they would drive up the whole group's premiums. And there is always the concern that the state medical board could take action that would affect the physician's license. A winning verdict is no consolation for the 2–3 years of their life that were wasted.

How can you get to a point where you accept the process as simply a game of strategy, like a chess match? We get to that place differently. It may take many lawsuits before it happens. But it does eventually happen for most.

A good model for how this process occurs is outlined below. It is based on the Elisabeth Kübler-Ross model describing the five stages of grief as written in her book, *On Death and Dying*. Not everyone goes through all five stages, but everyone goes through at least two.

Kübler-Ross stages of grief as a model of the pain from a medical malpractice lawsuit
- denial
- anger
- bargaining
- depression
- acceptance

Denial

Kübler-Ross definition
Denial is a conscious or unconscious refusal to accept facts, information, reality, etc. relating to the situation concerned. It is a defense mechanism and perfectly natural. Some people can become locked in this stage when dealing with a traumatic change that can be ignored. Death of course is not particularly easy to avoid or evade indefinitely.

Application to getting sued
When you hear of being sued for the first time, you are numb. You feel like you have been sucker-punched. And you do not know what to do. That is the reason for this book—during this stage you are very vulnerable and need direction.

Frequently, after the initial shock of getting sued, the physician denies the gravity of the situation. Perhaps, the physicians are so convinced of their innocence that they assume the case will simply "go away." Although their lawyer may tell them this is unlikely, the doctor refuses to face reality. As a consequence, they ignore their responsibilities as a client and fail to listen to their attorney's advice.

Another scenario has physicians in denial about a bad case, for example one in which there is obvious malpractice or where no expert will give testimony to defend their actions. Perhaps their attorney has recommended settling, and the doctor is insisting on going to trial.

Meeting with your (hopefully) compassionate attorney often helps you acknowledge your situation and deliver you out of denial. In fact, good attorneys can have the dual role of psychiatrist in addition to their legal duties. However, some physicians are very resistant. They are very stubborn and often refuse to exit this stage. Unfortunately, there are many physicians in this situation, and it can be very detrimental to their case. Doctors in denial are loathe to take any advice. Those who do not take advice can harm their case before it even gets going.

Anger

Kübler-Ross definition
Anger can manifest in different ways. People dealing with emotional upset can be angry with themselves and/or with others, especially those close to them. Knowing this helps keep detached and nonjudgemental when experiencing the anger of someone who is very upset.

Angry physicians make poor defendants.

Application to getting sued
Many doctors I speak to about previous lawsuits are still angry. Thus, this stage takes a long time to move through. Some are still angry at the time of trial.

What are they angry about? Obviously physicians are angry about being sued. But the issues can be more complex. Physicians may be angry at the patient for suing them and at the plaintiff's attorney for accepting the case. They are likely angry at "the system" for creating a situation that can disrupt their life and their practice.

Most often, however, physicians are angry at themselves. On some level, they blame themselves for doing or not doing something that would have prevented the bad outcome that led to a lawsuit.

Wherever you direct your anger, if you are not careful, you will jeopardize your performance at the deposition and trial. Being angry can prevent you from thinking clearly. If a jury perceives this, it can prejudice them against you.

Physicians need to present a calm and controlled appearance to the jury. A loose cannon will appear as just the kind of physician who would be likely to commit malpractice. Remember, in a courtroom appearance is everything. You must reconcile the anger you feel to project an ideal defense.

To that end, anger management is critical. Certainly, having constructive outlets to vent and deal with your anger, such as family and friends, can help. One of the most beneficial means of overcoming your anger is through discussions with other physicians who have been sued and survived. Although this may seem to conflict with the earlier advice about not discussing the case with anyone other than your attorney and spouse, it is not. You can certainly discuss your feelings of being sued, and learn from the experiences of others in the same position, without revealing details of your own ongoing lawsuit. Some physicians require professional help. Do not be ashamed to seek counseling. It can be a career-saving measure to do so.

Bargaining

Kübler-Ross definition

Traditionally the bargaining stage for people facing death can involve attempting to bargain with whatever God the person believes in. People facing less serious trauma can bargain or seek to negotiate a compromise. For example, "Can we still be friends?" when facing a breakup. Bargaining rarely provides a sustainable solution, especially if it is a matter of life or death.

Application to getting sued

I do not think that overt bargaining with a higher power is as much an influence in this situation. However, there often is something to that effect with your "higher self." For instance, you may make a promise to yourself, "I will be a better person/doctor if this case goes away."

The bargaining extends to their practice of medicine, "If I practice defensive medicine, then I won't get sued and have to go through this ever again." You think of all the ways of avoiding a lawsuit, and you do not deal with the issues at hand. You convince yourself that these changes will make you a better and more insulated physician. Although this stage does not necessarily have as much harm to your current case, it can act as a distraction. And it hinders your getting to accept your circumstances.

Depression

Kübler-Ross definition

Depression is also referred to as preparatory grieving. In a way it is the dress rehearsal or the practice run for the "aftermath," although this stage means different things depending on whom it involves. It is a sort of acceptance with emotional attachment. It is natural to feel sadness and regret, fear, uncertainty, etc. It shows that the person has at least begun to accept the reality.

Application to getting sued

There is a bright side to feeling sad all the time. It means that you are in the final stage of grief.

I know many physicians who are on the brink of tears for weeks or months at the very thought of their case. Their fears and frustrations are very much at the surface, and they have trouble keeping them bottled up. Clearly, this lawsuit is affecting them on a very personal and emotional level. However, if these emotions show through when you are in court, once again, it can be devastating for your case. The jury will wonder about your competence if you are welling up with tears while at trial.

> Feeling depressed is normal. And it means you are well on your way to full, healthy acceptance of your circumstances.

Once again, having a support system to get you through this stage is essential. Your attorney often plays a crucial role in guiding you at this time by giving you critical confidence in your case and in yourself. Once you can reconcile the self-pity you feel as a result of the frustrations of the lawsuit process, you will be a stronger person and better physician.

Acceptance

Kübler-Ross definition

Again this stage definitely varies according to the person's situation, although broadly it is an indication that there is some emotional detachment and objectivity. People dying can enter this stage a long time before the people they leave behind, who must necessarily pass through their own individual stages of dealing with the grief.

Application to getting sued

The key is, "emotional detachment and objectivity." As physicians, we try to practice medicine this way to ensure the best treatment of patients with devastating conditions. It does not mean we do not care, but the objectivity is key to making clear decisions.

When dealing with the emotional trauma of a lawsuit, the same credo applies. In this case, you are in the final stage of acceptance when you tolerate your circumstances. You may not like it, but to heal you must acknowledge that being sued is part of the cost of doing business. Only when this occurs are you best able to act on your own behalf. Knowing the rules of the game, you are now ready to play to win.

Nobody said it would be easy. In fact, the process is very difficult. There is always a temptation to regress into denial and anger. And even physicians who successfully move through all the stages do not necessarily avoid the practice of defensive medicine. Efforts at tort reform have lowered premiums but have not been proven to reduce this common reaction to the possibility of being sued.

There is another psychological model, by Abraham Maslow, that helps explain why physicians who under normal circumstances act in an altruistic fashion change their behavior under threat from a medical malpractice lawsuit. This model is explained in both his article, *A Theory of Human Motivation*, and his book, *Toward a Psychology of Being*. He postulates in his writings a needs-based hierarchy of human motivation and behavior.

> The Maslow model's five stages of needs can explain why defensive medicine occurs, and how hard it is to eliminate this practice.

The basis for his theory is that human beings are motivated by unsatisfied needs, with the lower, more basic needs having to be satisfied before the higher, more selfless needs can be actualized. The first four needs, beginning with the most basic, are the *deficiency* needs that must be fulfilled for a person to act unselfishly: psychological, safety, social, and esteem. In other words, if you do not have enough of something, you feel the need, and thus the motivation to fill it. A given person must complete these before moving to the highest level of need: self-actualization. According to Maslow, if a person feels threatened, nothing higher in the hierarchy will receive attention until that need is resolved. Below is a brief description of each stage:

1 *Psychological*: breathing, food, water, sex, sleep, homeostasis, and excretion. These are the basic needs of existence and form the building blocks

for life. Unless these essentials are met, nothing further on the scale of motivation can be recognized.

2 *Safety*: security of body, of employment, of resources, of the family, of health, and of property. This next stage seeks to avoid physical and emotional harm. Here people are guarding their resources. In another sense, you become concerned with your fears and anxieties and attempt to create order and structure as a result.

3 *Social*: also called the love/belonging need, deals with friendship, family, and sexual intimacy. This is the first of the higher needs, as the focus shifts outward from self to the interaction with others. You seek a sense of community and may try working in a group or team.

4 *Esteem*: self-esteem, confidence, achievements, respect of others, and respect by others. Once a person has a sense of belonging, the next evolution is the need to feel important, and have pride in their work.

5 *Self-actualization*: morality, creativity, spontaneity, problem solving, lack of prejudice, and acceptance of facts. Maslow felt this was the peak of the hierarchy of needs, and the point at which individuals can realize their full potential as a human being. People in this stage are usually seeking more meaning through truth, justice, and wisdom. However, according to Maslow, only a small percentage of people reach this stage.

Under stressful conditions, people can regress to a lower need level. Maslow postulated that if you have significant problems somewhere along the hierarchy, you may fixate on those needs for the rest of your life.

This model explains physician behavior very well. Beyond the basics of physiological needs, physicians seek security. Thus, they have a house, life insurance, disability insurance, medical malpractice insurance, and health insurance. Physicians, for the most part, have experienced monetary adversity for a large number of years, creating the *deficit* that Maslow describes. Thus, they are motivated to counteract that with their higher income and creation of assets.

The physician's working environment is very much a team, including the nurses, physician extenders, receptionist, and of course, the patient. Thus, the physician is motivated by social needs. However, if physician reimbursement keeps getting cut, while their medical malpractice insurance costs more, and their 401K keeps going down, it may be very difficult for the physician to continue being a team player. Thus, the physicians may begin acting disagreeable to their spouse and coworkers and spend less time with their patients.

Likewise, if the working environment breaks down to the point that the physicians cannot trust their colleagues and their patients, it is unlikely you can do much to motivate them to achieve the "best practice" goals that the government recommends (an example of the next need level, *esteem*). Physicians need strong support to get to a point where they are motivated solely by seeking pride in their practice of medicine. Finally, physicians cannot actualize the idealistic vision of medicine they imagined as a medical student (the fifth need—self-actualization) unless they have a strong sense of self-confidence.

> Deficiency of a need leads to the motivation to fill it—for physicians, financial security and self-esteem are the largest drivers of defensive medicine.

On the basis of my interpretation of Maslow's observations of human motivation, physicians who are sued will likely suffer a breakdown in the second stage of the need for safety and security. Physicians will enact asset protection plans, increase their insurance limits, and suffer extreme anxiety at the thought of losing everything. They may obsess about maximizing reimbursement. At this point, the physician's priorities change to the lower needs. And as long as they continue to regress away from self-actualization, they will look at life differently than before. They will practice medicine differently than before. They will abandon their intuition and their compassion. Their altruistic practice of medicine will cease to be a motivating factor until the physician is able to reconcile these fears.

Those that manage their safety need can still be stuck in one of the next levels of motivation. It is here where the practice of defensive medicine begins to be ingrained, either from a lack of trust of their colleagues, team, or patient (*social* need) or from a lack of trust in their own abilities (*esteem* need). Regardless, once fixated on these deficiencies, it is hard to break free to advance to a point where your sole interest is in taking care of the patient.

If you use Maslow's supposition that only a small fraction of humans are self-actualized and apply it to physicians, then unfortunately, only a small percentage of physicians will be practicing selfless, compassionate medicine. In addition, those physicians that have reached the pinnacle of motivation can become frustrated when forces outside of their control (e.g., administrators or HMOs) demand that they practice in a manner that conflicts with their ideals.

> Threats to security and confidence trigger the Kübler-Ross stages of grief. Moving into acceptance will eliminate the feelings of deficit.

To relate this to the aforementioned Kübler-Ross model, the physicians who have been sued are hit at many points in their basic needs hierarchy simultaneously. The threat to financial security and self-esteem are too much for even the most altruistic physician to handle. Thus, they experience the stages of grief as mentioned by Kübler-Ross. Once the physicians have moved into acceptance of their circumstances and eliminated the feeling of deficit that Marlow describes, they can once again move up the hierarchy to the higher needs and the selfless practice of medicine. But as I said earlier, the more traumatic the deficit, the longer it will take to resolve the feelings of loss.

Strategies for coping

How does the physician successfully move into acceptance? Time, as always, is a key to healing. And as mentioned earlier, having a good, sympathetic attorney helps. Most importantly, having a strong support system of friends, family, and colleagues will make it easier to get through this as well. Listed are five strategies for coping:

1 *Pay attention to your attorney*: They have had many clients in your situation, and they know how to best bring you through the process.
2 *Focus on your case*: If you concentrate on the particulars, there will be less uncertainty and thus less anxiety.
3 *Be objective*: The emotional detachment you use to practice medicine effectively is well applied to your malpractice case.
4 *Learn to play the game*: I know this is your life, and it does not seem like a game, but a lawsuit has opponents who use strategy to prevail. You need to learn the rules and play to win.
5 *Ask for help*: From your friends, from your colleagues, from your family, from your attorney, and from a psychiatrist if necessary. Do not let your problems coping ruin your case and harm your career.

If you are resistant, it may take a long time for this healing to occur. However, it is vital that you do everything possible to move toward a resolution of these stages of emotional healing, which are a natural reaction to being sued. Sometimes the advancement of your case through the legal process can be the trigger that is required. The time period after you have been sued is fraught with fear and uncertainty. Taking each stage in a step-wise fashion, without panicking, can help a great deal. Chapter 5 discusses in more detail the critical period that is between receipt of the initial complaint and the pretrial deposition.

Chapter 5 **Before the deposition**

By this point, you have passed through the initial shock of receiving the summons, and you have chosen an attorney. The first topic on the agenda will be addressing the complaint. There is a limited time to answer the complaint, and you will need to speak with your attorney within a few days of receiving notification of a lawsuit against you.

Soon after being served, you will speak with your attorney:
- Were you legally served?
- Was the case filed in federal or state court?
- Now your complaint will be addressed so that your attorney can get enough information to formulate a response.

Were you legally served?

Your attorney will want to know how you were served to see if it was a proper service. For instance, if you never received it personally either directly or indirectly through a third party, and the only summons you received was by mail, it would not be proper. Your attorney will also want to know if this case is within the statute of limitations; thus, they will likely ask you what the dates were that you rendered care for this patient. You will need to fax a copy of the complaint to your attorney so that they can fully evaluate these issues.

Was the case filed in federal or state court?

Another important item in the complaint that your attorney will be very interested in evaluating is whether the case was filed in state or federal court. The majority of medical malpractice lawsuits will be tried in state court. In fact,

---

How to Survive a Medical Malpractice Lawsuit. By © Ilene R. Brenner. Published 2010 Blackwell Publishing.

so few cases are tried in federal court that most medical malpractice attorneys will never try a case in that venue.

However, I did mention in Chapter 2 that cases that have Emergency Medical Treatment and Active Labor Act (EMTALA)-related issues can be tried in federal court because EMTALA is a federal statute. Thus, there are many differences between the two venues (http://uncivillitigator.blogspot.com/2005/05/federal-versus-state-court.html). The federal court may have different and stricter evidentiary rules from most states. These are the regulations that govern what facts get considered or precluded from consideration by the court, jury, or arbitrators to determine whether the substantive conditions of liability are satisfied. These rules govern what testimony, documents, photographs, recordings, and the like are admissible and what weight should be given to particular evidence admitted (Anderson 2005).

The most important of these requirements demands expert testimony. Federal court uses what is called the Daubert standard for expert witnesses, which is a series of stringent expert requirements in scientific cases. Many states have loose requirements as to who can be defined as an expert, and thus, trying a case in federal court enables the defendant in one of those states a more favorable legal environment (further details on experts and the Daubert standard are given in Chapter 7).

Another difference of federal from state court is that federal judges have paid law clerks and interns working for them. This allows more time and resources for thoughtful and thoroughly researched contemplation of motions than state judges, who rarely have more than an unpaid intern assisting them (see Chapter 8 for more information on what a motion is and why you might want your attorney to make one to help get your case dismissed).

Most of the rules in federal court seem to favor the defendant. However, different jury panel makeup under state court and federal court rules can alter the strategy. A jury panel is a list from which jurors for a particular trial may be chosen. There could be higher or lower concentrations of individuals with an ethnic background, which could serve to favor the plaintiff or defendant. A typical federal jury pool is much less diverse, with fewer minorities, as it represents registered voters in a federal district, whereas state courts have county residents for their pool. In cities and other cultural diverse areas in particular will have this distinction as registered voters statistically have a lower percentage of minorities than occur in the local population. However, many rural areas will be less culturally diverse, and therefore, there will be little difference in the jury pools. There may be issues of race that might favor the plaintiff using the federal jury panel. However, it is more frequent that state court jury panels will have concentrations of plaintiff-friendly people, and thus, incentivizing plaintiffs toward using state court as their preferred venue.

Another example of why a plaintiff might want to file a case in federal court is if your locality is known to be tough on plaintiffs. In this situation, the attorney would have an incentive to move the case out of state court.

What kind of cases typically find their way into federal court? If the parties involved in the case are from different states, the federal court system would likely be available to the patient, provided they have the requisite jurisdictional amount of $75,000. This is a common reason in medical malpractice cases as patients often visit physicians from out of state. Another reason to move a case to federal court would be if the case involved federal statutes such as EMTALA (as was discussed earlier in Chapter 2).

More often than not, there are many differences between federal and state court statutes. Thus, it is imperative that you *insist* on an attorney that is experienced in trying medical malpractice cases in federal court. As very few medical malpractice lawsuits end up in federal court, there will not be many defense attorneys with the requisite experience. Do not accept an attorney who has not tried cases in federal court as the variability from state laws could put you at a disadvantage (see Chapter 3, *How do I change my attorney?*, for more information on this critically important topic). The insurance company has a duty to provide an experienced attorney to best defend you.

Addressing the complaint

Of course, your attorney will want to know your opinion of the allegations made against you. At this early stage, you may not have had enough time to be able to get all of your records. If the patient was seen in an office setting, you probably have easy access to the records. However, if the patient spent any length of time in the hospital, you might not be able to get a copy of the records without the official requests from your attorney. Therefore, in attempting to give your opinion of the complaint, you likely will not have much documentation to reference.

Assessing your case will be much simpler if you have a strong recollection of the patient. Obviously, it will be easier to do your evaluation if you have a complete office/hospital chart, and you take time to review any other notes or insurance forms that could have information not found elsewhere. However, with the large number of patients a physician sees, it is possible that you will not be able to add much through your own recollection. If physicians have no memory of the patient, they need to obtain a copy of as much of the patient's chart as is possible and give opinions based on what is written in the chart. Once your attorney has as much information as you can provide, they will put together your denial to the complaint.

The discovery phase begins

Attached to your answer to the complaint are formal legal papers that include a demand letter that begin the discovery phase of the lawsuit. The demands are usually for different kinds of records. After you have spoken with your attorney, he or she will have enough insight into the various defense scenarios that are being considered. However, in all likelihood, he or she is probably not looking beyond the immediate issue of answering the complaint. You should not be too concerned at this point if you are not formulating your defense.

In the next step, in some jurisdictions, your attorney waits for the HIPAA authorizations to arrive. Those are then mailed out to the various doctors and hospitals. Later on in the litigation process, as you near trial, your attorney will issue trial subpoenas and trial authorizations. In other states, the subpoenas for records are immediately issued. At this point, not much happens while your attorney waits for records to be delivered. The attorney and their staff review those records in detail. You will receive copies of any records you do not already have that were created by you or the nurses/staff working with you. You usually will not receive records of subsequent treating physicians because the more you read, the more that could be asked about later on in the deposition (see Chapter 6 for more information about the deposition).

Sometimes, the prior or subsequent treating physicians are reluctant to release their records for fear that they could be brought into the case. If this occurs, your attorney will need to issue a subpoena, and a notice to take a deposition of that physician, to obtain these records. Essentially, your attorney will be forced to take a deposition on a physician just to obtain information essential to your case. Usually this is not necessary, but it does occur.

> Discovery: Not much seems to happen from your point of view, but your attorney is receiving and assimilating a huge amount of information critical in the defense of your case.

Meeting with your attorney

A few weeks prior to your deposition, you will have your first face-to-face meeting with your attorney to begin to prepare you for what is one of the most critical parts of your case. At this meeting, your attorney may ask you to do some relevant research for your case. Any research you do at this point is protected by attorney–client privilege. This is the stage where you start discussing strategies for your defense.

The first attorney meeting is very important to the physician's psyche because this is the first time the defense strategy will be addressed. The first few weeks after you find out you are being sued are likely the worst moments because of your feelings of helplessness and uncertainty. These meetings with your attorney give you a partner to guide you through the process of making concrete plans that go a long way to alleviate your frustrations and anxieties.

The inhouse physician review

At this stage, you will want to have as much information as is possible, and you might have access to an inhouse review that is conducted at the behest of the insurance company. In this situation, the insurance company has physicians on staff who review your case file. Although these reviews can bring to light important issues relevant to your case, they may be of limited value to you, the physician, as these reviews are not done at the request of the attorney, but at the request of the insurance company. Thus, the reviewers are employed by the insurance company and may be biased toward the insurance company's interests. These reviews can be done for a high-exposure case to determine whether the insurance company should consider settling the case, and can also be done randomly as part of the insurance company's periodic review. It is usually done before depositions, and can be re-reviewed after the depositions to see if the case should settle or go to trial.

As this assessment goes over defense issues, it is possible that the reviewer could recommend settling a case that the attorney (or you) thinks is winnable. The attorney has no say at this point, and it is left up to you, the doctor, who has the *consent to settle* clause in their insurance policy, to refuse to allow the insurance company to settle a winnable case (see Chapter 8 for more information on this critically important topic). Therefore, the inhouse review can lead to tension between the physician and the insurance company. Unfortunately, if you do not have the clause in your policy, your insurance company is well within their rights to use the reviewers' comments as basis for settling your case.

As reviewers use hindsight in assessing your case, they may miss or misinterpret important points that led to their decision to have your case settled. If you feel they erred, whether you have the *consent to settle* clause in your policy or not, give a detailed and thorough written rebuttal to your insurance company with a request for another review. Do not come off angry and bitter in your rebuttal. Just stick to the facts. Most insurance companies will consider your request.

Although it would be helpful to have an expert's opinion at this stage of your case, most insurance companies will not approve the hiring of experts until all plaintiffs and defendants have been deposed.

> The inhouse reviewer could recommend settling your case even though your attorney feels it is defensible. The *consent to settle* clause in your policy is your only protection from this.

Rejecting a settlement request to progress the case

At some point, you will likely be confronted with an offer to settle your case. Although this usually occurs after the depositions are taken, it can happen at any time, even while the jury is in deliberation. In some states, a rejection of a settlement that becomes a plaintiff's verdict can result in penalties against the physician. In those states, the initial settlement offer is simply a procedural issue to take full advantage of a law that says that a plaintiff can recover interest on a proposed settlement amount that was rejected by the defendant(s). The purpose for this is to encourage more settlements and discourage unnecessary use of the court system. Thus, this initial request is usually for a ridiculous sum, in the anticipation that the offer will be rejected, especially if the plaintiff senses that the defendant(s) wishes to take this case to trial. It is a way for the plaintiff's attorney to set the stage for increased damages (see Chapter 8 for more information on settlements and Chapter 10 for more information on damages). Again, having a clause in your policy that allows you to have the final decision in regard to settling your case is the ideal situation. Once you have officially rejected a settlement, the process of scheduling depositions occurs. More information about deposition is provided in Chapter 6.

Reference

Anderson RE (2005) *Medical Malpractice: A Physician's Sourcebook.* Humana press, Totowa, NJ, p. 17.

Chapter 6 **Nail the deposition**

The most important part of your case is upon you—the pretrial deposition. If you do a poor job, you can ruin your case and make a defensible lawsuit become indefensible. What is a deposition? It is the sworn testimony of a witness taken before trial, in a location that is out of a court setting, without a judge present. Still, the witness is placed under oath, a court stenographer records the testimony, and if necessary, translators will be present.

It is the practice in most states that the plaintiff and all defendants have depositions taken before trial. In addition, there may be a deposition of the plaintiff's spouse. Some states permit the deposition of experts and some states do not (see Chapter 7 for more information).

The deposition process consists of meeting with plaintiff's attorney face to face while they question you for as long as it takes in an attempt to lock in your testimony and to try to prove their case. The plaintiff's attorney can then use what you say to frame questions at trial. Contrary to what you may think, the deposition is rarely for your own benefit. It is not there to clear up the facts so that the plaintiff's attorney can realize just how wrong they were for suing you.

There is a common misconception among physicians that if they explain things well, their intelligent responses will prove to the plaintiff's attorney that the whole thing is a mistake. They may also think that they need to explain their defense clearly and completely to the plaintiff's attorney. However, as will be detailed later on in this chapter, a general rule is, "the less you say, the better." Because there is the potential to do significant damage to your case, it is critically important that you perform well; otherwise, you may be forced to settle an otherwise winnable case.

> The deposition is not there to help you convince the plaintiff's attorney to drop the case against you. It simply locks in your testimony for trial.

How to Survive a Medical Malpractice Lawsuit. By © Ilene R. Brenner. Published 2010 Blackwell Publishing.

Preparing for the deposition

Your first step in your preparation is to meet with your attorney to explain the process

Some attorneys hire trial/jury specialists to help you. Often, attorneys supplement their own preparation with these experts who get you ready for your deposition and trial. If you are given the opportunity, use it. If not offered, ask if this is possible.

Few attorneys spend the time and effort required to make sure you are "ship-shape." If your attorney does not prepare you adequately for your deposition, you will likely perform poorly (especially if this is your first time). A preparation expert can fill in the gaps and give you the extra confidence you need to do a great job at the deposition and trial. I have found that even if it is only one or two things they tell you that help you, it is worth it.

Know your strategy for dealing with codefendants

At the time of the deposition, all codefendants should be cooperating with each other. Even if you think one of your codefendants committed malpractice, this is not the time to mention that fact. Keep that information to yourself until backed into a corner where you have no choice but to reveal that. Why? You do not want to help the plaintiff's case at all.

> Form a united front with your codefendants and try not to point the finger at them.

You might think that revealing this information might get you out of the case leaving only the "true guilty party." Wrong. Turning on your codefendant will not help you get out of the case. In fact, it will likely ensure your staying in the case because your codefendants' finger will now be pointing directly at you. Thus, you will fall into the trap set by the plaintiff's attorney; sue everybody in sight and have them turn against each other so as to get money from at least one of you. Work with your codefendant(s) and provide a united front. Do your best not to say anything that could make the other look bad; however, of course, make sure that whatever you say is within the confines of truthful testimony.

If you have a corporate entity, such as your boss's company, as a codefendant, it is to your advantage to do and say anything your attorney recommends to help get them dismissed from your case. For instance, if you have independent contractor status, there are legal tactics that can show that your boss is in no way tied to any possible medical malpractice on your part. Although this may seem like you are getting the shaft in favor of your company, it is to your benefit to separate yourself from them. This is an important part of your case, as jurors like to award money to plaintiffs when a corporation is involved. The last thing you want is to have jurors in a mood to award money.

Make sure you understand well the basic medicine components to your case

If you are wrong on the medicine, it will not matter what your defense is. All may be lost and you have not even started the trial. Now that you have met with your attorney (as opposed to before), go ahead and do your research and make sure you have got the medicine correct. Your research is protected by attorney–client privilege, and thus, is not discoverable by the plaintiff's attorney.

Be aware of subsequent treating physician testimony/ documents, but DO NOT read those documents yourself

I know on the surface that this does not make much sense. However, think about what I just said about less is more. The more you have read before the deposition, the more you can be asked about.

There are many circumstances where knowing information about subsequent treating physician testimony/documents can be helpful to you. For instance, in the instance of a heart murmur, you might not have documentation that specifies heart sounds. It is likely you do not remember if you heard one or not. However, if asked if you heard a heart murmur, you might be inclined to say "no," because it was not specifically charted. If you were to then find out that the cardiologists who saw the patient subsequent to you all heard murmurs, you might want to finesse your answer so as not to look incompetent. In this case, it would be better to simply say, "I might have, but it is not explicitly documented." Sure, this shows you did not document your examination perfectly, but it prevents you from saying something that is clearly opposite to subsequent expert physicians.

So how do you know what is in documents you never read? That is where your attorney comes into play. Your attorney will read those documents. And they can inform you of any information they deem important. That way if asked if you have any knowledge of subsequent treating physician testimony or documents, you can say, "only what my attorney told me." Boom! Attorney–client privilege is now brought to light. The question is objected to, and you cannot be asked about anything that your attorney told you.

Choose an appropriate location

Your attorney's office is the best place to have the deposition. But it really can be at the courthouse, plaintiff's attorney's office, or in any conference room. Do not host the deposition in your office or hospital as anything in there, such as diplomas, books, or journal articles, could become fodder for questions by the attorney.

What should you wear to your deposition?

You should look clean, neat, and professional. Nothing flashy. You should look, "put together," like someone who will make a good impression with a jury. You would be surprised how many physicians disregard this basic rule. In fact, I have heard of many instances where the physician puts up a big fight to try to get out of dressing nicely to the deposition. Yes, it is stupid. Yes, it is superficial. Are you going to lose your case because you decided to wear jeans and a T-shirt to the deposition? Not necessarily.

However, you might end up going to trial on a case where you might previously have been dropped. This is because some plaintiff's attorneys sue everyone in sight and use the deposition as a fishing expedition. If the plaintiff's attorneys think you will come off poorly on the stand, they may keep you in the case hoping your poor performance will make them money.

Thus, the need to dress nicely is not to be underestimated. At a deposition, you are being judged by your words *and* by your appearance. The plaintiff's attorneys are watching you closely; do not give them anything with which to find fault. Although you do not have to wear a suit, you do want to look sharp. If that means buying a new outfit for the occasion, then do it. That extra expense pales in comparison with the consequences of a lost medical malpractice lawsuit.

Tips to nail the deposition:
- get as much training as possible
- know your medicine
- dress appropriately
- treat the questions in a business-like manner

The plaintiff's attorney

Every lawyer has a different style. Some like to talk a lot. Some give speeches. Some pretend to be super nice. Others are confrontational. Your lawyer can often have insight as to the style you should expect. Regardless of the tactical style of the plaintiff's attorney, your mission is the same: to remain calm and answer questions with thoughtful consideration.

At the deposition

No matter who the plaintiff's attorneys are, there are some general rules that you need to follow for a successful deposition.

Treat the questions in a business-like manner

Be polite. Answer the questions as succinctly as possible. And never parry or be sarcastic with the plaintiff's attorneys. Do not be funny. It does not come off well on paper. Just play it straight, cool, calm, and professional.

More deposition tips:
- be confident
- do not interrupt the questioner
- use "medicalese" generously
- the less you say, the better

Be confident

If you have insecurities, they will come out. Make sure you go over the case with your attorney until all of your doubts about your case go away. Make sure you can defend anything but offer nothing unless asked. You need to strike the right balance between confidence and arrogance. If you are at the deposition stage, you have made a conscious decision to take this case to trial. Of course, information could come through the depositions that can change whether or not the case actually proceeds further.

However, you are going into the deposition with the knowledge that your treatment was within the guidelines of good and acceptable practice. There should be no doubts in your mind about any issues in this case. If you present a strong front, the plaintiff's attorney will realize that you will also make a formidable opponent on the witness stand. Your good performance in the deposition could lead to your being let out of the case (especially if you have other codefendants who give a weaker appearance).

On the contrary, if you are arrogant, the plaintiff's attorney will realize that you are the type of doctor who has the kind of personality that will turn off juries. Any chance you had of getting your case dismissed will likely be gone.

Do not accidentally let out how busy it was in the emergency department

If your case involves the emergency department in some manner, it is not to your advantage to describe a frenzied scene. Those types of comments open you up to comments about how little care you gave to this patient. Although it may be true that it is commonly known that emergency departments tend to be chaotic, busy places, you should not reiterate this fact. The show E.R. among others has helped create this image. However, words such as "chaos" and "busy" are easily linked to words such as "error" and "mistake." They expect your department to be busy and do not consider this a viable excuse for the patient's poor outcome. Also, jurors like to imagine themselves in your emergency department, recreating the incident. You want them to imagine a pristine environment where only the best medical care is delivered.

Lab values: know your acronyms

Oftentimes, you are asked about the lab values. If you are asked to give your opinion on the CBC, do not just hit the highlights. Go through each element, including the mean corpuscular volume (MCV), in excruciating detail. Also, make sure you know what MCV and other less commonly used abbreviations stand for.

For instance, you might be tempted to say, "The patient had no anemia, and a slightly elevated white blood cell count." However, you should give many more details than are expected, "the white count is barely elevated at 14, the MCV is normal, the MCH is slightly low, the MCHC is normal, the left shift is barely elevated at 76, the eosinophils are normal ..." Do you get the point?.

Why is this important? The plaintiff's attorney is trying to focus your attention on the critical values in the case. They want it to appear that the whole CBC is abnormal. If you only hit the major points of abnormals in the CBC, you will fall into their trap. However, if you give every value in the CBC, likely some things will be normal. These normals especially help your case if your CBC is being used to compare to a previous or later one.

For instance, there could have been a previous CBC a few days prior that had a normal white count, a normal left shift, a low hematocrit, low MCV, low Mean Cell Hemoglobin Concenration (MCHC), and normal Red Cell Distribution Width (RDW). If your CBC has an elevated white count, an elevated left shift, a normal hematocrit, normal MCV, normal MCHC, and normal RDW, now on a comparison basis, your CBC is actually slightly improved overall.

If in a case about infection you hit the highlights of the significant abnormals, in other words, just focus on the white count and neutrophil count, your CBC will appear to be worsened overall compared to the previous one. On an open-ended question like this, you have the power to make your CBC appear in a better light than simply pigeonholing two key values. Neither is a right or a wrong way to present the CBC. However, one clearly is superior in its interpretation. It is the difference between getting forced to admit that your CBC is abnormal compared to previous and being confident in your defense that your CBC is actually slightly improved. Look for other ways to turn an apparent weakness in your case into a strength. However, if you are asked directly about only one particular value, make sure to simply answer directly to that one value. Providing extra information as above could appear disruptive.

Do not interrupt the questioner
Every word said can affect the meaning of a question. Do not interrupt, as it looks rude and can cause you to answer incorrectly.

It is a natural inclination to want to make the attorney look foolish and to show how smart you are. But do not do it
You are on his turf, and you will lose. Do not speak in a condescending manner to the attorney. Even though you may be tired, frustrated, and annoyed, answer the questions in a straightforward manner.

Use medicalese generously
In other words, try to use specific medical terminology and jargon wherever possible. This is an excellent strategy to force the attorney to use their medical knowledge. Some attorneys are smarter and better prepared than others. If the plaintiff's attorney does not completely understand your answer, it is harder for them to formulate questions to counteract it. Therefore, you should force the plaintiff's attorney to use their own knowledge and experience to devise questions.

Sure, the attorney could make you explain what you just said. But most attorneys have egos, and constantly having you explain your answers to them will make them look stupid. You would be surprised at how many attorneys would not follow through with a line of questioning just because they do not want to look stupid.

For example,

Say, "… distal to the MCPJ in a circumferential pattern …"

Do not say, "… just beyond the first knuckle that makes a circle around the finger …"

When answering questions beware of certain traps:
- rule out
- double negatives
- compound questions
- statements that precede the actual question
- hypotheticals

Beware of "ruled out" in a question

Q: Did you *rule out* appendicitis in this patient?

This is a very tricky question. We as doctors use the term "ruled out" very differently than the layperson. Do not assume that the attorney means it in the same way.

A: What do you mean by "rule out?"

Make the attorney give their own definition of "rule out" and then answer the question in that context. Chances are that they will bounce the question right back to you.

Q: Why don't you use it in the context that you would as a physician?

Now is your opportunity to define it yourself, so that it is very clear.

A: I generally define the medical term "rule out" as "a diagnosis is not consistent with the overall presentation of a patient."

These small things can help (or hurt) your case a lot. For instance, if you had simply accepted their definition, your line of questioning could look like this:

Q: Did you *rule out* appendicitis in this patient?
A: To the best of my ability.

Q: Did you do a CT scan?
A: No.

Q: So then how can you say you ruled it out?
A: The patient did not require a CT scan.

Q: Are you aware that the plaintiff did in fact have appendicitis?
A: Yes.

Q: Is a CT scan not commonly used in the diagnosis of appendicitis?

The plaintiff's attorney will continue in this fashion, until they tell you that you "missed" the diagnosis of appendicitis. You will control the flow of questions much better if you get clear definitions for apparently simple phrases.

By the way, in case you are asked if you "missed" something, as before with "ruled out," make sure to ask, "what do you mean by missed?"

Beware of compound questions

If a question has two or more parts, do not answer it. Your attorney should object to this question. But if that does not happen, you must state that you cannot answer because there are multiple questions being posed in that question. Ask for a breakdown so that you can answer one part at a time. MAKE SURE YOU KNOW EXACTLY WHAT QUESTION YOU ARE ABOUT TO ANSWER.

Example

Q: What would have been going on between 1900 h and 2100 h? Would the patient be monitored by the nurses during this time?

In this case, it is two separate questions compounded together. But the effect is the same. You are tempted to answer both. You should make them break it apart into separate questions, "I'm sorry. Could you rephrase so that I am only answering one question?"

Beware of questions that are preceded by statements

Sometimes, the plaintiff's attorneys will speak one or more sentences before asking an actual question. Beware of these situations, because you may not realize it, but by answering the question, you may have, by implication, agreed to the statement they just made.

Therefore, if a question is preceded by a statement, wait for the end of the statement/question, then ask for clarification as to what the question was. Do not get sucked in by this common tactic.

Example

Q: Looking at the values on the overall hepatic function panel, there were four findings that were elevated. To what did you attribute those elevated levels in the hepatic function panel?

In this case, you must be sure that the attorney is accurate in his or her assertion that there were four abnormalities. Maybe there were five abnormalities. Or two. The plaintiff's attorney might be making an innocent error, or might be trying to trick you. Regardless, try not to answer these questions. If you do, listen to the statement very closely to make sure you agree with it before answering the actual question.

Beware of double negatives

Sometimes a plaintiff's attorney will inadvertently (or purposefully) confuse you by asking a question that contains a double negative. You may think you understand the question, but before you know it, you have answered it wrong.

Example

Q: It is my understanding that not stabilizing the patient is an EMTALA violation. *Isn't it true that the patient was unstable upon transfer to the other hospital?*

This is where keeping it simple can actually hurt you. If you answer with a simple "yes" or "no" as advised earlier in the chapter, you might answer "no" when you mean "yes." For instance, in the above example, you likely will answer "no" to the question.

When you hear that question in conversation, it seems like a simple question because your ear ignores the contraction as a negative. When you read the question, and then separate the contraction to "is not," the double negative becomes apparent. Because all double negatives cancel out, the question *actually* says, *Is it true that the patient was stable upon transfer.*

Now, your answer is clearly, "yes." So which is it, "yes" or "no?" Good question. Therefore, avoid these issues by going into further depth or by making them restate the question.

A no. 1: Yes, the patient was stable upon transfer.

A no. 2: I do not understand your question.

or

A no. 3: I cannot answer yes or no the way you have phrased it.

One trick to recognizing double negatives is to listen for a contraction or the word "not." Also, any question that begins with "Did you not …" should never be answered. Pay close attention to words that by definition are negative because of two letters: for example, *un*stable, *im*material, and *in*ability. If you hear any of these in a sentence, get it rephrased.

Do not guess

It is alright if you do not remember. Simply say, "I don't recall." Even though it may seem monotonous, you will not look stupid even though it feels strange to say those words over and over. Do not offer what you "could" have been thinking or even what you "should" have been thinking.

> Do not let the attorney pressure you into giving an answer when there is not one.

Sometimes the attorney, after a few "I don't recalls," will try to corner you.

Q: Now that you have reviewed the chart, the labs, and so on, what do you now think the patient had?

Again, your answer is the same.

A: I can't answer the question because I don't know what my thinking was at the time. The chart doesn't help me improve my recollection.

They may push harder.

Q: Let us just say you saw this patient today, under these same circumstances, what would you think?

This is where most doctors fold and start offering up opinions. Your answer, again, is the same.

A: The presence of a patient is critical to making accurate diagnoses, and therefore, I cannot make any suppositions as to what the patient could have had, given that limited example.

A good plaintiff's attorney will take this one step further, and they will turn it into a medical school type question.

Q: If a patient presents with fever, SOB, and tachycardia, what is part of your differential diagnosis?

The trick here is to answer as broadly as possible, give them 10 possibilities. If your case is about a missed PE, don't say, "Well, it could be PE."

A: It is a very long list of conditions that meet those criteria.

Make the attorney work for it. Do not make their life easier. Make them counter with.

Q: Okay, please give me that list.

Do not answer hypotheticals

As indicated earlier, sometimes the attorney will ask you a hypothetical question about a general patient encounter. This point is so important that I wanted to separate it out into a separate section. Only answer questions that relate to *this* patient in *this* case.

The less you say, the better

Do not teach the plaintiff's attorneys the facts. Let their own experts do that. Think of it this way: the deposition is a document that is going to be used against you. The less there is, the less harm there can be. And as physicians, we are taught "do no harm." Therefore, abide by that motto when preparing for the deposition.

The following are two series of exchanges between plaintiff's attorney and doctor, with the same information.

Exchange no. 1:

Q: Do you speak Spanish?

A: I speak Spanish for medical purposes. I can maybe make my way in Mexico or Spain a little bit. But I can get a history and a physical on about 90% of my patients independently. On occasion, I will ask for a translator if I find it necessary, like for discharge instructions. I am better at speaking, and understand if Spanish is spoken slowly. I remember talking with my patient in Spanish, and understood what was said to me. However, I did get a translator to give my detailed discharge instructions.

Exchange no. 2:

Q: Do you speak Spanish?

A: Can you be more specific? Do you mean am I fluent or do I speak *any* Spanish?

Q: Do you speak Spanish with your patients?

A: Yes.

Q: Do you ever use a translator?

A: Sometimes.

Q: Under what circumstances would you use a translator?

A: While I will occasionally require a translator for obtaining my history and physical, I mostly use one for explaining the discharge instructions.

Q: Did you use a translator with the plaintiff?

A: Yes.

Q: Do you remember what you used a translator for?

A: Yes. I used one to give my detailed discharge instructions.

As you can see from the above two exchanges, there is a clear difference in how the same information comes across on paper. The first exchange is more conversational. And although that may seem more natural, on paper it appears less clean and professional. It also opens the door for lots of questions that you may think are irrelevant but can become a long tangent.

For instance, you can now be asked questions about your medical Spanish, like "Did you take any courses on medical Spanish?" or "Have you ever traveled to Mexico or Spain?"

And those questions will lead to more questions, and before you know it, you have spent half an hour or more with tiring questions that have little to do with the actual case. These questions wear you down, so that when you do get to important questions, you are more likely to slip up.

Upon reviewing the second scenario, you can see how by giving minimum information, more questions were generated, but they were more specific. Less leeway was given to come with more questions. It is a much better way to exchange information in a deposition setting. Also, note in the second exchange, the doctor answered the question with a question. Not only is this acceptable, but it is also a preferred method of making sure you are answering the "right" question.

Sometimes what you think the question is saying is not clear. As I just mentioned above, you should never guess. If it is not overused, asking questions is an excellent way to distract the attorney, probably to get a clear question to answer. The plaintiff's attorney wants to ask more general questions that get you to say more. You want to give specific answers to specific questions. Thus, asking for clarifications can help break down a general question into two or more specific ones.

Do not think that if you say something it will suddenly end the questioning

As I mentioned earlier in this chapter, the more information you give to the plaintiff's attorney, the more questions they will think of. And do not think that anticipating their next question will save time either. It will only give them five more questions to ask you.

If you do not offer any details, they will have to work harder and may forget to ask things. After all, they do not know the medicine as well as you do. Therefore, unless you trigger their memory, they may forget to ask something.

The goal is to force the attorneys to supply their own knowledge during the questioning process. Because you have forgotten more than they will ever know about medicine, this is clearly to your advantage. If they ask you a question where they clearly do not know what they are talking about, do not go out of your way to teach them the medicine.

Example

Q: When you gave toradol, a very powerful medication for pain, you simply covered up the symptoms but did not actually treat the patient?

A: That is not an accurate statement.

Make them try to figure out what part of that was inaccurate. They made the mistake. Make them fix it. Do not help them. Do not tell them that toradol is no stronger than motrin (save that for trial). Do not tell them that toradol can cure inflammatory processes as it is an anti-inflammatory medication. Also, do not tell them that treating pain is essential to the care of the patient, ethically and according to JCAHO.

Do not go into a long explanation after saying no or yes

No means no, and yes means yes. Do not give an explanation instead of saying no or yes.

Example

Q: Do you remember how many times you visited with the patient?

A no. 1: No, it could have been two. Maybe three. I did not document it, and therefore, I am not sure. I usually check on a patient at least three times per shift.

Bad answer.

A no. 2: No, but I usually check on a patient at least three times per shift.
Better answer.
A no. 3: No.
Best answer.

Exception to the "less is more" advice

There might be a circumstance where your attorney could tell you on a "bathroom break" that for one specific issue you should explain things more in depth. However, leave that to your attorney's discretion. As a general rule, you should not assist the plaintiff's attorney. However, there may be one or two core issues where clarification *may* result in a dismissal of the case.

For instance, let us just say, during the deposition, it is clear from the plaintiff's attorneys' questions to you, that they do not understand a critical issue in your case. They might not understand that there is a difference between a neurologist and a neurosurgeon, and they cannot understand why a neurologist would not come into the hospital to clip an aneurysm. If the attorney understood the difference between the two subspecialties of medicine, your previously negligent appearing actions might be revealed as correct.

The following scenarios explain the previous statements more clearly.

Q: Doctor, did you call in a neurologist to fix this patient's aneurysm?

There are two scenarios here: the limited answer and the answer with some explanation. Usually you would choose the less is more tactic. However, look at how this plays out below to see why, on occasion, in limited use, a detailed explanation can greatly help your case (or even help it get dismissed).

Scenario no. 1:
A: No.
Scenario no. 2:
A: No, a neurologist is not a surgeon and therefore would not be the correct specialist to call. In this case, a neurosurgeon is required.

If you simply answered like in Scenario no. 1, it is possible that you just reaffirmed the plaintiff's whole reason for suing you: you failed to call in a neurologist. However, if you answered like in Scenario no. 2, you answer the question, but you explain why not calling a neurologist was not negligent. Now you have helped your case significantly. Or, at the very least, helped counter one of the plaintiff's issues against you. In summary, only answer to what you are asked, as briefly as possible. Use your attorney as a guide to know if there are certain issues you should explain in more detail.

Other things to do at the deposition

Take breaks!

Bathroom breaks. Soda breaks. Lunch breaks. This gives you an opportunity to converse with your attorney and adjust your tactics as necessary. And it helps you recharge a little bit, as being at a table full of people while someone asks you a barrage of questions can be very tiring.

> Taking breaks allows you to recharge and strategize with your attorney.

Assume that everything is on the record!

If you are on a break and speak with your attorney, it must be behind closed doors. You do not want the plaintiff's attorney to have extra ammunition against you. Also, when you are in the deposition room, even words casually spoken with others in the room outside of questioning may be recorded. Be very careful not to say anything.

This advice is not limited to what you say. You also must be careful of anything you bring with you into the deposition room. For instance, if you have notes or make notes during the deposition, the plaintiff's attorney is well within their right to ask you about what you have on the papers in front of you. There was a situation in my deposition that happened to end up working in my favor in this regard.

Before my deposition, my attorney gave me a little note that said that new information was recently uncovered about the plaintiff that simply said "DUI" with a date. This was a tremendous development in my case as alcohol abuse by the patient was part of our defense as an explanation of the patient's uncommon presentation and severe complications. Rather than toss the note in the wastebasket (which I should have done), I stuck it in my folder that was brought into the deposition. At the end of deposition, I started getting many weird questions about my drinking habits, criminal history, and so on. Eventually, the plaintiff's attorney admitted that the reason for this line of questioning was that he could see from my notes (he read them upside down from across the table) that there was a DUI. My attorney interrupted and said, "that's your client."

> Do not be upset if your attorney is friendly with the opposing attorney. It is part of their strategy. Ignore it.

When the deposition is over, LEAVE THE BUILDING QUICKLY!
Do not hang around to talk with your attorney later. If the plaintiff's attorneys think of another question, they might call you back into the room. They cannot do that if you are not there.

Clearly, the deposition *can* make or break your case. And if you have a good case to begin with, you may even get lucky and get your case dropped or dismissed. If not, you will at least set yourself up well for your trial. Another critical component of your case is the expert opinions that will probably support your defense. How do you pick the right expert? Chapter 7 has more on this very important topic.

Chapter 7 **All about experts**

After the depositions of the plaintiffs and defendants, your attorney (and/or the paralegals) will thoroughly review the records available and will send a copy of the complaint and the records to an expert they believe might be good for this case. Although your attorney might ask your opinion regarding certain aspects of the process of selecting experts, typically your attorney makes these decisions for you. For instance, they might ask your opinion about what specialists would be most/least appropriate to give expert testimony in your defense.

The most important part of your defense is being able to find a qualified expert who will support you in your claim that your care was appropriate and did not deviate from good and acceptable practice. If you cannot find an expert, you have no defense. To defend or prove a medical malpractice claim, the first issue that must be met addresses whether the physician's actions met the standards for good and acceptable practice (otherwise called "standard of care"). Thus, an expert is needed to declare what the standard of care is.

Some states require that the complaint be accompanied by a written testimonial, called an affidavit or certificate of merit, from an expert physician. If a proper expert is not used to certify the claim in those states that require it, the attorney can make a motion to dismiss on this basis (for more information on motions to dismiss see Chapter 10). Unfortunately, many states simply ask that any licensed physician can certify a claim against you.

There is also state-by-state variability on deposing the experts (giving testimony before trial). Some states permit that all experts for the defense and plaintiffs must be deposed before trial. Other states do not have expert testimony given until trial. In those states, the expert is not usually hired until late in the process to keep the element of surprise. It becomes much more important to quickly find appropriate experts in the states who depose

How to Survive a Medical Malpractice Lawsuit. By © Ilene R. Brenner. Published 2010 Blackwell Publishing.

them. Whereas in the other states, that decision could be held off for years, until shortly before the trial.

> It is a big advantage to be able to depose the experts before trial.

Also, this initial expert opinion is usually not the same person who will become the plaintiff's expert against you at trial. In fact, it usually is not, especially if you have your trial in a state where you do not depose experts. The plaintiff's attorneys will not want to reveal their expert in advance of trial to minimize opportunities to find information that could impugn their character or qualifications.

What qualifies a physician to be an expert?

This is subject to much variability. Some states are more stringent (and in my opinion more appropriate), requiring that expert opinions be given by physicians in your own specialty. I have listed in Addendum A all the states that have some version of the "own specialty" requirement. Others simply require knowledge of the subject at hand.

The problem with experts who are familiar with a specific topic but are in a different specialty than the defendant is that physicians in other specialties have a completely different perspective on what is expected in a given situation. For instance, surgeons cannot properly give an opinion on emergency physicians who missed appendicitis. Although they may understand well how to diagnose and treat appendicitis, they do not know or appreciate the difficult process that emergency physicians face when attempting to get the proper disposition for their patient who has vague or conflicting symptoms. Likewise, an emergency physician cannot judge the actions of a surgeon whose patient returns to the hospital emergency department with an abdominal abscess status post appendectomy.

> Qualifications on experts vary greatly by state.
> • Some require active practice and same specialty.
> • Some simply require an MD.

Some states such as Arizona are much more restrictive with language that specifies that to qualify as an expert in a medical liability cause of action, the physician must be licensed in the same profession as the defendant and maintain board certification in the same specialty of the defendant if applicable.

Plus, physicians must devote a majority of their professional time to the active clinical practice or to instruct students in the same health profession as the defendant for the year immediately preceding the occurrence giving rise to the lawsuit.

Other states such as Alaska require that experts be licensed, trained, and experienced in the same discipline or school of practice as the defendant. However, their qualifications could simply be directly related to the matter at issue. In other words, some states determine experts not based on having similar qualifications as the defendant but on their knowledge of specific issues in the case.

To complicate matters further, some medical malpractice cases are tried in federal court (see Chapter 5 for more information about federal versus state court venue), and those lawsuits have very stringent expert requirements that are called Daubert rules based on a 1993 Supreme Court case *Daubert v. Merrell Dow Pharmaceuticals, Incorporated*. In this case, the Supreme Court ruled that cases with scientific evidence are determined by the expert testimony and the court must act as a gatekeeper to determine whether the testimony is scientifically valid and applicable to the facts at issue (Reeg and Bebout, 1997).

Daubert rules regarding medical expert testimony: three questions must be answered

1 *Is the medical expert qualified?*

An expert should be a treating physician with personal knowledge of the plaintiff's injury and history. Some courts further require that there be appropriate specialization to diagnosis and treat the plaintiff's injury or disease.

2 *Is the medical testimony reliable?*

Many factors go into this estimation, which is usually where the specific requirements most dramatically deviate from most state courts. For instance, testimony is considered reliable if the plaintiff's expert has personally examined the patient as well as reviewed all the medical records (this is exceptional as no state has this stringent of a requirement to be an expert—see Appendix A). An expert should employ standard scientific practice by performing objective tests, using medical assessment technology, to formulate a differential diagnosis, develop a working diagnosis, and rule out alternative causes.

Most importantly, the expert should not form the opinion first and then go in search of facts to support that opinion. The experts' testimony will be suspected if they have not conducted independent research on the subject matter outside of the lawsuit. Federal courts have rejected the testimony of the experts who have arrived at testable conclusions but have not tested those conclusions and subjected them to scientific scrutiny. In other words, the "hired gun" who is willing to testify on just about anything will not survive analysis under *Daubert*.

3 *Is the medical testimony relevant?*

Essentially, the expert testimony must include much more than general statements of fact relevant to the case; it must establish "specific causation."

For example, in a case involving treatment for hyperbilirubinemia (Sartore and van Doren, 2006), experts often state "with reasonable medical certainty" that performing additional phototherapy or an exchange transfusion at an arbitrary level of total serum bilirubin would probably have prevented a neonate from developing kernicterus (bilirubin-induced encephalopathy). However, there is a paucity of medical literature that establishes the relative risks in this specific situation. Thus, a *Daubert* motion to bar expert testimony could be made successful because it cannot be proven based on the medical evidence that the negligence could have been the cause of the damages (a motion is a legal procedure that brings a limited contested matter before the court for a decision).

There is much in medicine that is performed as the standard of care but is not overwhelmingly proven by the literature. An expert cannot testify that you committed medical malpractice if clear scientific evidence that shows the relative risks regarding the specific issues in your case has not been established. This is a critical distinction of the *Daubert* rules compared to typical state court laws.

The *Daubert* hearing

A hearing is a legal proceeding in front of a judge. A *Daubert* hearing would be scheduled before the trial to judge the appropriateness of expert testimony. The court's role is limited to determine whether the proposed expert's testimony is derived from an application of the scientific method and "fits" the issues in the case. The hearing provides an opportunity to preview the opponent's case.

Obviously, it would be impossible to have a hearing without speaking to the expert and documenting their testimony. Therefore, as in many states, the experts are deposed before trial. As the plaintiff may win or lose based on the expert testimony, if the plaintiff's expert is precluded from testifying on an essential element of the case based on the results of the hearing, it is possible to make a motion for summary judgment to get the case dismissed (see Chapter 8 for more on this topic). Sometimes the defense attorney will make this motion *before* the *Daubert* hearing; hence, the court may review all the issues at one time, in other words, decide whether the expert testimony is appropriate *and* whether issues of fact exist to warrant a trial in an effort to get your case dismissed earlier and faster (http://www.mobar.org/journal/1997/novdec/bebout.htm).

The defense expert

Generally, your expert will be an MD not a DO. (This varies by location as some areas of the country understand the equivalence and others do not.) Experts will have great credentials: for example, board certified, experienced, Head of Department, published multiple papers. Typically, the most effective expert is published on the critical topics in your case. Physicians who are academics but keep an active practice are particularly valuable as experts.

One of the best qualifications an expert can have includes being on the specialty board that determines key rules on controversial topics such as TPA. However, *the* most important qualification is having a congenial personality.

> Aside from a great CV, charm is the best quality in a defense expert.

Your attorney cannot use physicians unless they are on the insurance company's panel. Of course, if the perfect physician experts for your case are not on the panel, attorneys can submit their CV and follow the appropriate procedures to get them approved. Not all attorneys do this. Some just choose someone on the panel. Unfortunately, if a physician has been an expert for many years, the juries can get an impression that physicians are simply a "professional expert." Therefore, using the same panel physicians can have risks. On the other hand, a physician who has the perfect qualifications and appears to have the perfect demeanor, but is not yet on the panel, is a risk. You never know how physicians will perform on the stand until they do it. If they choke, your case can be lost.

How many experts do you need? If at all possible, you need to have one expert. Insurance companies do not want to pay for multiple experts unless there are complicated divergent issues in the case that require expertise in two different specialties.

At trial, the defense expert is usually the last witness in the case. You want to leave a lasting positive impression on the jury, because this is the last testimony the jury will hear before he or she goes in to deliberate. When it comes to defense strategy, sometimes attorneys will hold back with your examination and of the plaintiff's witnesses on a critical issue in the case. This is done as a deliberate effort to reveal new testimony that the plaintiff's experts cannot refute. The only option left for the plaintiff's attorney would be to ask the court's permission to bring in a rebuttal witness; however, these requests are usually denied. The plaintiffs can then only make an attempt to repair the damage in their final statement to the jury; however, this is rarely effective.

What can you expect in a plaintiff's expert?

Again, although states vary, you can expect experts who are in your specialty. Their qualifications can vary greatly. They should and often do have top credentials. However, they often do not have much more than a confident demeanor and an inclination toward receiving large payments for giving opinions favorable to whoever writes the checks.

Sometimes the plaintiff will have multiple experts for different purposes. In complicated cases with multiple fields, it may be necessary to have an expert for each issue to address causation (the topic of proximate cause is addressed in Chapter 2). However, the plaintiff's attorney may have one expert who is there to speak to damages (i.e., make the case for a large award). Those experts usually have something specific in their background that will support the assertion of the need for a large monetary award.

Having multiple experts can be fraught with danger as having more than one expert on the stand increases the likelihood that they will say the same thing (in many states you cannot have two experts give repetitive testimony). Conversely, the experts might differ on an issue, and the conflicting opinions can confuse the jury and dilute the plaintiff's case.

If you live in a state where there are less stringent expert requirements, it may seem unfair and frustrating to see plaintiff's experts give testimony against you when they are not in your specialty. However, a skilled attorney can twist that around to work in your favor. For instance, your attorney when cross-examining the plaintiff's experts will ask them what field of medicine they are board certified. Then, your attorney will pepper the experts with questions about their training in your specialty. It will become clear to the jury that the expert is not trained in the same specialty as the defendant; a fact your attorney will reiterate during his final statements, "Why didn't the plaintiff's attorney produce an expert in the defendant's field of specialization? In this whole state they couldn't find one doctor in the defendant's specialty that was willing to give expert testimony against my client? So instead of producing an emergency physician, the plaintiff hires a family practitioner to fudge it? " Arguments along those lines can seriously damage the plaintiff's experts' credibility.

Also, some plaintiff's attorneys hire experts from outside the state. They may do this for many reasons, including getting a nationally renowned physician who may have written multiple papers on the issues in your case. It could also be that they could not find an expert in your state who would agree to speak on their behalf. Attorneys will point out in their examination of the experts that they are not from the state where the trial is being held and make some allusions in their final statement that states that the plaintiff could not find any physician in-state to defend their point of view. In some states, juries are particularly sensitive to issues of locality and may take offense that the plaintiff's attorney hired an outsider.

> It is not a tragedy if you live in a state with loose requirements. A good attorney will point out the inadequacies of the plaintiff's expert training.

What if the plaintiff's expert is not well qualified to give testimony against you?

A common way for defense attorneys to poke holes in the plaintiff's case is when they use the plaintiff's experts against them. When your attorney cross-examines a plaintiff's expert, the initial questions delve into the physician's qualifications. If attorneys can make it appear like their experts are not someone the jurors would trust to treat themselves, then whatever advice that they give will not carry much weight. Your attorney will fashion a line of questions that typically include:

Q: You gave testimony earlier that you attended and graduated from the University of Guadalajara in Mexico. Is this true?

Q: Your training in Mexico was not recognized in the USA without taking additional qualifying exams such as the ECFMG. Is this true?

Q: I noticed from your CV that you entered medical school in California and stayed there for one year. Is this true?

Q: Then there is a gap for the next year. Is this true?

Q: Then you went to a different medical school for the next three years. Is this true?

Q: Were you suspended or expelled from the California medical school, and what were the circumstances?

Q: You are not board certified in plastic surgery. Is this true?

Q: Did you fail to pass your specialty board examination or did you just not think it is important to take an exam that establishes basic standards for medical practice in plastic surgery?

Also, plaintiff's well-qualified experts can be used to help your case. If they are competent, truthful, and easygoing, the jury will be inclined to believe what they have to say. Although this might seem to be a big disadvantage from the defense's point of view, it is not so.

> A great defense strategy is to get the plaintiff's expert to agree to facts that are out of context but actually help your case.

This is one critical instance where an accomplished defense attorney can do a lot of damage to the plaintiff's case. Your attorney's goal is to structure the questions so as to appear innocuous and get the expert to agree with some apparently small issues of fact. Only later, during the defense's expert's direct examination, and again, during your attorney's summation, will these facts be placed in the desired context. Thus, it reveals the huge advantage the defense has in being last to present their case to the jury. When your attorney uses the plaintiff's expert's own testimony to support your defense, and that expert is very believable, it significantly helps your case. An example is as follows:

1 Plaintiff's expert is asked about the classic signs of appendicitis, and naturally states that anorexia is among them. Then the defense attorney gets the expert to agree that a hungry patient likely does not have appendicitis. Subsequently, the expert is shown an excerpt from the chart that reveals that the patient was hungry, asked for food, and ate. Defense counsel asks them to pin down when the patient could have perforated from appendicitis. Now they see the trap, but do not know how to evade it. Hence, the attorney continues by asking whether the hungry, eating patient had perforated. When they admit, reluctantly, no, then the attorney has now established, using the expert's testimony, that the patient must have perforated sometime after eating. Thus, the defense attorney has successfully used the plaintiff's expert to establish facts that helped the defense in this case.

2 A surgeon expert for the plaintiff is in court to give testimony for damages. However, on cross-examination, they are asked about what they feel causes sepsis in case of appendicitis. The physician states that the ruptured appendix is the cause of sepsis. The defense attorney make sure to get the surgeon to confirm that, indeed, you cannot have sepsis develop until the appendix perforates. Again, this fact helps the defense, but as it is out of context, the expert has no idea.

3 In their final statement to the jury, the defense attorney now puts together the facts as stated by the plaintiff's experts. You do not get sepsis until the appendix perforates, and you do not perforate if you are hungry and eating. This establishes the time course that the physician (the defendant) who treated initially could not have missed sepsis as the chart shows the patient being hungry and eating 24 h after seeing the physician. Although the defense experts may say the same thing, the more powerful words come from the experts who are inclined to disagree.

What if their expert is lying?

Obviously, it is frustrating for the defendant to watch calmly as the plaintiff's expert glibly lies about key facts in your case. Some of these experts obtain a large percentage of their income in a professional expert capacity. Therefore, they are very skilled at twisting around the facts and making misleading comments in an easygoing confident manner. Under these circumstances, it can be difficult for the jury to discern what is the "real" truth.

> Do not show to the jury your outrage if you think the plaintiff's witness is stating inaccuracies on the stand. It could backfire and make you look bad.

If you spot a lie that you think your attorney might not have picked up on because of the medical minutia involved, then casually, without emotion, jot something down on a notepad for your attorney. He or she might find it helpful during the cross-examination.

Again, this is where a skilled trial attorney makes or breaks your case. Your attorneys' job is to trap the experts in a lie they cannot talk their way out of. If they cannot show that the expert is lying, then the jury may believe these lies as truths. If your attorney can convince the jury of the expert's deception, then it will go a long way toward helping you win your case.

Another possibility is that your attorneys might think your information unnecessary and will stick with their original game plan. Do not get upset with them if this happens. They are the trial expert and see the big picture.

In the jury's deliberations, they must sort out the plaintiff's experts and the defense's experts and decide who to believe. If they feel the plaintiff's expert(s) misled them and distorted the truth, they will likely believe the facts from your expert and therefore decide in your favor.

I do not want to infer that all plaintiff's experts are liars as many of them are highly qualified with high integrity. However, some are so egregious in their distortion of the facts and arrogant for their successes in the past, they feel they can simply continue this practice without penalty. I am proud to say that I, in a small way, helped to out one of these physicians and would like to share the story:

A few years ago, an attorney whom I know was trying a case and was cross-examining a physician. Every time the physician was cornered in a lie, he would counter with another smooth lie. Most physicians, when trapped, have some visible sign of panic that indicates that they are not being truthful and get caught, but not this physician. His manner could not be shaken.

It was late in the day, and the attorney was questioning him about his hospital affiliations. He stated the hospitals where he had active privileges, and one of these happened to be the hospital where I had worked. This was an amazing coincidence because I live far away in another state. The attorney managed to convince the judge to finish for the day and allowed him to complete his cross-examination of the expert the next day.

Naturally, that night, the attorney asked me whether I knew this physician, but I had never heard of him. I called the head of the department to ask whether this particular physician had any privileges at the hospital. It turned out that the "expert" who was lying on the stand did not have privileges. He was supposed to have them, but for some reason did not complete the necessary paperwork. He also misrepresented his current whereabouts to his employer, who was very surprised to find out that while still receiving a salary to work, he was instead receiving additional money to be an expert.

The next morning, it was a simple matter to confirm with the hospital's credentialing department that he, in fact, did not have privileges to work at this hospital. Armed with this information, a trap was set where he would be asked again about his hospital privileges. When confronted with the fact that he did not have privileges and was giving false testimony, he again tried to lie his way out of it. Even the plaintiff's attorney was so horrified by his own expert that he asked the jury not to blame his client for his expert's testimony. The jury found for the defense, and the plaintiff's expert physician lost his job. Sometimes, what goes around really does come around.

At this stage in your lawsuit, the depositions are complete, the experts have been selected (and depending on the state, deposed as well), and all settlements are rejected. Now your attorney applies to have your case put on the trial calendar and you wait—what could be months or years for a trial date. Once you have one, you need to make preparations. More on this is described in Chapter 8.

References

Reeg KB, Bebout CK. What is all about, Daubert? J Missouri Bar 1997;53(6). URL http://www.mobar.org/journal/1997/novdec/bebout.htm.

Sartore JT, van Doren R. *Daubert* opinion requires judges to screen scientific evidence. Pediatrics 2006;118(5):2192–4. doi:10.1542/peds.2006-0052.

Chapter 8 **Pretrial countdown**

Here is your guide to pretrial elements you do not want to overlook

Review your deposition

First, you need to make corrections to your deposition. Although this might not seem like a big deal, it actually is. This is where you need to fix any transcription errors. However, there can be another use: fine-tuning a few key answers. Of course, states differ on this point, but many states will allow you to make corrections if you, for instance, misspoke.

> Make reviewing your deposition transcript a priority. Read it closely and correct inaccuracies.

Let us just say you answered something one way, and on reading the deposition you realize that you really meant to say something completely different. You got nervous and you said that INR means Internal Normalized Rate. You can fix that. You cannot change your whole testimony, but if you feel your answer as it appears in the deposition is not what you meant to say, then you can fix that. As your deposition is the most important part of your case, you want it to be as accurate as possible.

It should be noted, however, if the attorney for plaintiff chooses, he or she can try to confront you with an inconsistency by reading your original answer and then the correction to the jury. This could be embarrassing if you completely rewrote your deposition. Use this ability judiciously.

This is why, when your attorney sends you a copy of your deposition, you should not put it under a pile of stuff and forget it. You need to read every

How to Survive a Medical Malpractice Lawsuit. By © Ilene R. Brenner. Published 2010 Blackwell Publishing.

word, very carefully, and make your corrections. Again, states differ, but you can have as little as 60 days to submit your changes.

Besides your deposition, there will also be depositions of the plaintiffs and relevant family members. As mentioned in the previous chapter, in some states, you also depose the experts. In those other states, you will not know what the plaintiff's experts have to say about you until they give testimony at trial.

Once the depositions are out of the way, depending on the type of case you have, there may be an Independent Medical Exam (IME). For example, in orthopedic or neurological cases where the plaintiff is complaining of permanent disability, you will want to verify this with an independent physician. Also, in these types of cases, you will probably want to hire a private investigator as (I know this is shocking) plaintiffs sometimes lie about the true extent of the impairment to their activities of daily living.

Motions

There is a way that you might be able to get your case dismissed. The problem is that the success rate is low. Your attorney will probably hate me for even bringing up the subject. But here goes:

A *motion for summary judgment* is a method by which you can win your case without a trial. Your attorney will make this motion to a judge who will decide if the case does not have merits to proceed to trial. As mentioned previously, a motion is a legal procedure that brings a contested matter before the court for a decision. In this instance, the decision you want is to have the complaint dismissed.

> A motion for summary judgment cannot be made until all the depositions have been completed.

Reasons for making a motion:

1 The main reason is of course to get out of a case that you never should have been pulled into. I know, we all should not be in our cases. But still, there are some people who really should not be in a case. Those people might be let out of a case if the motion is successful.

2 If a motion for summary judgment is made, even if it is lost, it requires the plaintiff's attorney to defend the motion. This means that the plaintiff's attorneys have to reveal their strategy for the case, including the expert testimony they will likely use. This is a huge advantage for the defense to know this information. Also, it is costly as the plaintiff's attorney will have to pay his or her expert for an affidavit in opposition to the defense

motion (an affidavit is a written statement made voluntarily and confirmed under oath). To do this the expert will have to review the entire file.

So why doesn't everybody make a motion for summary judgment all the time? It is time consuming for the defense as well. If you know that there is little to no chance of winning, then the insurance company will be upset at a waste of their funds. More importantly, if the court deems the motion frivolous, then your attorney could be sanctioned with a fine of thousands of dollars. You should make a motion only if you have a good chance of succeeding.

Could you win a motion to dismiss?

What kinds of situations warrant a motion? This is a tough question. Technically, your case must have no issues of fact to decide. This is legalese and hard to grasp, so ask your attorney if you have reason to make a motion. As a quick example, if you had seen a patient who had compartment syndrome from a cast placed the previous week, and he or she has sued everybody involved including you, then you might have a case that would be good for a motion.

Another situation is mentioned in Chapter 7, regarding the *Daubert* rules for federal court expert testimony. These rules can be invoked to block the critical testimony of the plaintiff's experts who are essential to proving the "facts" in the case. Thus, if the experts are denied, and no other evidence exists to support one or more of the required elements of its cause of action, there are no issues of fact to decide and the case cannot proceed to trial.

What if I think my case would be a good one for a motion, but my attorney disagrees?

First, you need to ask yourself, is my attorney acting in my best interest? That goes back to the previous chapter describing *conflict of interest*. Do you have any codefendants who might be influencing your attorney's decision?

If you have co-defendants, it is possible that making a motion to dismiss you from the case could help you at the expense of your co-defendants. If you are in this situation, you have a classic case of "conflict of interest." "That is the clue that it is time to ask for a new attorney, so he can make the motion and represent your interests."

If you do not have codefendants, and you did your due diligence in choosing good attorneys, then trust them. If they say your case is not right for a motion to dismiss, then accept the decision and move on. You can still win your case at trial.

Settling your case

Should you settle?

At this point in your case, all the information is out on the table. Your insurance company and your attorney now know the true risks and benefits of going to trial. It is at this point where the question of settlement could be raised.

Again, according to the specifics of your insurance policy, you may or may not be allowed to have the final say on this very important decision. This is why, and I will mention it once more to reiterate the point, you must try to get the "consent to settle" clause into your medical malpractice insurance policy.

> The consent to settle clause gives you control over whether to settle the case or not.

Any advice I give regarding settlement is possible only if you have the final say. If your insurance company and/or your employer have this control, you are at their mercy. And if you are in this situation, you might end up settling a very winnable case because they forced you into it. Some mention of the topic of settlement has been given in Chapters 1–3 and 5. However, I will be going into much more detail at this time.

What are the benefits of settling out of a case?

1 You have an indefensible case.
   • *What is an indefensible case?* A case where no expert witness is willing to testify on your behalf.
2 You have a defensible case that can go for more money than your policy covers you for and can put your assets at risk.
3 Psychological benefit of not having a medical malpractice lawsuit to worry about.

> There can be advantages to settling:
> • high exposure cases that could go over your insurance limits
> • psychological benefits of ending your case

What are the benefits of NOT settling?

> Doctors win nearly 80% of the cases that go to verdict.

1 As physicians win the majority of cases that go to trial, your odds are very good (AMA website, medical liability reform fast facts

http://www.ama-assn.org/ama1/pub/upload/mm/399/mlr_fastfacts.pdf—is
actually referenced from Physician Insurers Association of America, 2005).

2 If you settle for more than approximately $10,000 (this varies in each state
   and with each insurer), then your insurance company will surcharge your
   medical malpractice policy.

3 Too many settlements can lead to a policy surcharge, or even an inabil-
   ity to perform certain functions such as surgery. A surgeon who is not
   allowed to operate likely will not be able to maintain their previous standard of living.

4 Depending on the state you live in, too many settlements can trigger the
   state medical board to investigate you (refer to Chapter 2 for more information about the state medical board). You definitely do not want this. It
   is the quickest path to lose your privilege to practice medicine.

5 Any payment for even as low as one penny made by your insurance carrier will thrust your name into the National Practitioner Data Bank.

6 Plaintiff's attorneys often sue doctors because they want a settlement.
   They want the easy money. It costs them a lot of money to take a case
   to trial. Therefore, if fewer doctors settled their cases, plaintiff's attorneys
   would need to be much more selective in picking which patients they will
   take on as clients. More selectivity equals less lawsuits overall.

> Once you are in the National Practitioner Data Bank, it is permanent. This is a
> key point to realize when you are settling for what seems to be an insignificant
> amount of $1.00 (which can happen in states such as New York because of
> peculiarities in the law that were actually designed to decrease the number
> of lawsuits that go to trial).

So what should you do?

- If you have a defensible case, it may be better to lose at trial than to lose
  by handing over the plaintiff easy money. Better to make them work for it.
  (Caveat: You must ensure that it is a case that will not exceed your policy
  limits.)
- If you have a defensible case, you are more likely than not to win your case.
- It is best to keep the settlement option on the table for the time you get hit
  with an indefensible case.
- Use your option to settle judiciously. Take all of your cases to trial if you
  have a defensible opinion from an outside expert and adequate insurance
  coverage limits.
- However, what do you do if your case is defensible but high exposure? You
  might have to settle to protect your assets and home. This is a personal
  decision that only you can answer.

Take most cases to trial. You want to reserve the option to settle for when you get hit with an indefensible case.

The pretrial countdown

When your case is a few months before the trial date, you will want to be thinking about pretrial preparation. This is when you get serious about your case.

Become the expert

Read everything you can on the topic. Know all the statistics off the top of your head. Know every part of the medical record backward and forward. Study your deposition thoroughly.

This is why your deposition was so important. You need to go through your testimony word for word, line by line. You need to find anything that could be used against you, and identify something positive that will allow you to defend it and turn it into an asset. You should try to anticipate your weakest links, and what you may be asked on a cross-examination. You need to know the deposition so well that the plaintiff's attorney cannot trick you by quoting something out of context from the record (they will).

When you prepare for your trial date, identify your weaknesses and make them strengths.

Get as much coaching as possible

You will receive preparation from your attorney, and oftentimes, a preparation expert. They will assess you for your strengths and weaknesses. They will give you sample questions, so that you become more comfortable with the process. They will tell you what is expected of you in court. You may even have a videotaped session. This can be very much valuable, so that you can see your demeanor. Do you look nervous? Arrogant? Smart? Professional? Do you have annoying mannerisms?

Also, a preparation expert can help you look at your answers from a different perspective. I remember in my case I had very poor documentation for the history. And being aware of that affected how I was answering questions. The preparation expert showed me how I actually answered all the relevant information, just not necessarily in its designated spaces on the form. Once I realized that my documentation was not as bad as I thought, my answers were more certain. Confidence is the key. Any insecurities you have about your care or your chart *must* be resolved before you go to court. The pretrial preparation period is the time to work out these issues.

Preparation is everything. You need to be ready for battle. Trials are war. Coming in second does not cut it. It is your career on the line. You are your own best or worst witness. And Chapter 9 teaches you how to be the finest one possible.

Chapter 9 **The trial**

The process of getting sued for medical malpractice and heading into a trial can remind you of a Kafka novel. It likely has been years that the case has been somewhere in your mind, but now it is ALL you can think about. If your trial is within the next month, then you are probably getting little sleep, are eating either too much or too little, and are meeting all the criteria for generalized anxiety disorder. This is normal.

Everyone panics before his or her first trial. A million scenarios run through your mind, all bad. I know it is scary seeing your career flash before your eyes. A jury of your peers will soon decide your fate. This lack of control over your own life is unsettling at best and terrifying at worst.

> It is normal to be nervous, fearful, and full of anxiety as your trial date approaches.

The best advice I can give is focus on the endgame. Although the past few years of your life being dragged through the legal system may not seem like a game to you, it may help to view it that way. We all know that the legal system does not always dispense justice. He or she who has the better prepared attorney has the best chance of success. There is definitely a chess-type strategy that gets played out before and during the trial.

So what is your role in this game? You need to stop playing defense and begin playing offense. Suppress your anger and ego. Listen to your attorney. If you are careful to pick knowledgeable and experienced representation, do not flush your whole case down the toilet by ignoring their sage advice. Their reputation as trial attorneys hinges on winning as many cases as possible. They want to win. Therefore, pay attention to what they say. The little details that may seem stupid to you are likely more important than you realize.

How to Survive a Medical Malpractice Lawsuit. By © Ilene R. Brenner. Published 2010 Blackwell Publishing.

> How to be a star defendant:
> – keep your ego in check
> – listen to your attorney
> – keep your cool and be professional at all times

What are the rules to follow?

This is a little tricky to define, as the rules are somewhat different depending on what state and local customs dictate. Nevertheless, the commonalities and differences are worth noting.

How to dress

Professional. Clean. Like you are going to the most important interview of your life (you are). Some lawyers espouse a brand new suit every day of the trial. Others say a suit everyday, for a woman, is not necessary. In some parts of the country (or even specific counties within certain states), not wearing a suit to court is considered unprofessional. Other locations might find this pretentious and overdone. Thus, consulting your attorney for their opinion is imperative.

For multiple-week trials, have 1 week of unique outfits, and adjust the shirts/blouses/ties the following week with the caveat that you are in your best outfit on the day you appear on the stand.

Women must pay attention to what shoes they wear. Jimmy Choos are no more appropriate than Birkenstocks. Is it ridiculous to assume that a case will be sunk by the wrong shoes? Shoes that are inappropriate could place you in a negative light in the mind of a juror and create a subtle bias against you.

For similar reasons, leave the fancy jewelry or Rolex watches at home. For women, a nice set of pearls (fake is fine) will do well. You should not appear too glitzy, but you also should not look like today is just any day.

When to show up to court for trial

Local customs dictate whether it is appropriate or necessary for a doctor to attend jury selection (see the following text for more information on selecting a jury). In some locations, neither plaintiffs nor defendants attend. Some attorneys like to see the potential jurors (called a panel) through your eyes as well as theirs and want you to be present.

Others feel your attendance could turn off jurors before the trial even begins. And by being there, you might feel inclined to give your opinions that your attorney does not necessarily agree with and does not want to hear.

In regard to showing up for the actual trial, there are different viewpoints on what should be done. Some attorneys tell you to show up every day. Others will tell you to attend only certain days of the court. There may even be regulations that require you to attend all or certain days of the trial. For instance, it is nearly universal that you be in court on the day your case opens, the day you testify in court, and for all summations and the court's charge to the jury. Therefore, these decisions are best left to your attorney.

In the courtroom, you are under a microscope. The jury sees every twitch you make. Some lawyers believe that the more a doctor is in court, the more opportunity there is to give off a negative appearing facial expression and poison the jury against him or her. Therefore, those attorneys prefer their clients to attend as little as possible. Others have discovered that juries notice the plaintiff attending every day and feel that the defendant (you) should attend as well. Each scenario is valid. It is best to do whatever your attorney feels is most appropriate.

Jury selection

As mentioned earlier in the book, a jury panel consists of a group of people from which a jury will be chosen. The prospective jurors are then questioned in court by the attorneys—a process called *voir dire*. Sometimes judges who can ask questions themselves and address any controversy are present. In some states, judges are not present. The questions can be more general and asked of the entire pool and answered by a show of hands. As an example, the plaintiff's attorney might ask the panel if anyone might have difficulty being impartial with a gay plaintiff. In my case, my attorney jokingly asked if anyone would have trouble being impartial knowing that I grew up in New York (the case was tried in the south). Skilled attorneys (and their assistants, if applicable) will use these general questions as an opportunity to read the nonverbal language of each potential juror. What they do not say is often just as important as what they do say. Any jurors left after these general questions can then be subject to individual questioning, especially if the nonverbal language indicated that more information was needed.

The goal of the questioning is to find reasons for which a juror might become disqualified to sit on a jury. The US Supreme Court restricts the removal of jurors purely on the basis of race or gender. Both plaintiff's attorney and defendant's attorney also have challenges that allow them to remove a person from the panel without needing to give a reason. Because there is a wide variability on the number of jurors that can get selected for trial, there is also variability in the number of challenges each party can receive.

> Your attorney will ask prospective jurors questions to find reasons to disqualify them without having to use a challenge.

Sometimes the attorneys make an agreement that all people of a certain type will be disqualified to avoid wasting challenges and speed up jury selection. For instance, in a medical malpractice case, an agreement might be made to automatically remove all attorneys, physicians, nurses, and spouses of physicians.

The stated goal of questioning in jury selection is to see if they are able to follow the law and be fair and unbiased. However, when asked this, many people will make claims that they can be impartial when they actually are not. In reality, all people have preconceived opinions based on their life experiences. It is a clever attorney who can ferret out these hidden biases. Attorneys skilled in jury selection will do more than simply pick a jury. They will also plant the seeds to crucial issues that will come up at trial.

> The lawsuit trial begins in jury selection, and issues of the case may be addressed at this early stage to create subtle bias toward your case.

The trial of a case begins in jury selection. Your attorney wants to get the message across to the (potential) jurors that no matter how serious the injury is, you cannot decide for the plaintiff unless duty, breach, proximate cause, and damages exist (these topics are covered in Chapter 2). The question may be asked by your attorney, "If the plaintiff only proves some but not all of the essential criteria for a successful lawsuit, can you separate this out and find for the doctor? The judge will explain the law to you, can you follow what the judge tells you?"

Many attorneys go a step further and address critical issues in the case to desensitize the potential jurors. In medical malpractice cases, there is often a very sympathetic plaintiff. Following is a sample defendant attorney statement to the potential jurors meant to mitigate this common situation:

> "The plaintiff will talk a lot about sympathy. However, sympathy can be looked upon from a different angle. Sympathy is not simply an isolated emotion. It is joined by four other concepts: duty, responsibility, justice, and fair trial. If you decide this case solely on sympathy, then one of the parties in the case, whether plaintiff or physician, will not get proper justice, and someone will not be getting a fair trial. Can you assure me that you will lay sympathy aside when deciding this case?"

The attorney takes out a pen, "On the subject of sympathy, what does this pen have to do with sympathy? This pen is a tangible physical object. The pen is a 'fact' and has nothing to do with sympathy. Sympathy isn't an object; it is an emotion that we feel. I will ask you, I will put this pen on top of this ledge of this platform. Throughout the entire trial, visualize this pen. Whenever you feel sympathy, look at the pen and say that you will decide this case on the facts, not on sympathy."

This plants ideas with the potential jurors that the plaintiffs may have a high-damages case that they might not be able to prove. It preconditions them to look closer at the issues of breach of duty and proximate cause. It teaches the jurors how to be objective even when they want to be sympathetic. This is clearly to the defendant's benefit.

Opening statements

This is where both sides present their case. The plaintiff's attorney will lay out his or her case and what he or she intends to prove. Your attorney will then speak to deny that you committed any malpractice. Often, this is when the jurors decide who wins. It is scary to think that they have made up their mind so early in the process, but it happens. Often.

> The trial is like a roller-coaster:
> – The plaintiffs build their case against you.
> – If the early stages of the case appear to go badly, do not worry, it should.
> – After the plaintiff's crescendo, it is all downhill as your attorney makes your case and builds the momentum in your direction.

Plaintiff begins the case

The plaintiff's attorneys have a number of options for bringing people to the witness stand. They have their client, their experts, other relevant witnesses, and you.

Yes, you are a big part of their case. If you play it smart, you can diminish your part in the buildup of their case (more on this later). Oftentimes (and some would argue that it should be all-times), you will be the first witness to be questioned by the plaintiff's attorney.

Looking at the trials objectively, the plaintiffs' case begin at a high point. They get to say all kinds of bad things about you. But little by little, your attorney will chip away at their cases. The higher they start, the better for them. Therefore, they will often lay out their cases beginning with you, at your most vulnerable point. Their hope is that you will be nervous and an easy prey in their experienced hands.

Plaintiffs' experts and witnesses will say many things that will support their case. Understand this: you will not win every point. In fact, you will lose many points. However, look at it like a football game. It does not matter who leads at halftime. The winner is determined by who plays best in the second half. If you manage to win any points in the first half, you should feel very good about how things are progressing.

The cross-examination

As was just mentioned, the most common scenario is your cross-examination by the plaintiff's attorney during the plaintiff's case—typically, with you as the very first witness. However, it is possible that it could be later, after your direct examination by your attorney. The decision is at the discretion of the plaintiff's attorney. Your cross-examination could "make you or break you," and therefore, do your homework and nail it. Here is how you can do this.

First, there are several basic methods of cross-examinations. The ways you can respond are numerous. No question has a simple answer, and some may be designed to trap you into an answer that may not be wholly true. There are laws in each state that can restrict what you, the defendant, can say in response to a question.

The limited response

Some states insist that you answer with one of the following: "Yes," "No," and "I don't understand, I can't answer your question as phrased." In other words, you are prevented from giving details. If you try and say, "Yes, but that was because …," the attorney will object to strike everything after the word "yes." (Strike means to have testimony removed from the permanent record and to be disregarded by the jury.)

If you cannot give explanations, then you might think this a boring and pointless exercise. But plaintiff's skilled attorneys can fashion a line of questions that make you agree with them or disagree with them for a specific purpose. You, likely, will not see that purpose until it is too late. Do not try to anticipate this too much or you will overthink and harm your case.

Even if it seems like you are clearly making statements that make you look bad unless you explain things, do not worry about it. Just answer honestly. Your attorney will (if he or she gets to call you first) do a preemptive strike by addressing any possible issue in detail so that the jury already understands why you did or did not do whatever the issue is in your case. Or, if the plaintiff calls you first (the most common circumstance), then your attorney can fix any "damage" by going into each issue in detail when he or she has the opportunity to ask you questions.

No matter who calls you to the stand first, there is always another chance for both plaintiff and defense to question you again. This is called a re-cross and re-direct examination. It is a tactic where you are questioned again to make a point not made previously or to "fix" any poor answers you may have just given inadvertently. However, this strategy should be used sparingly, if at all.

Juries often perceive a re-direct or re-cross as a damage control effort (which it is). They know that any issue brought up at this time must be very important, and therefore, they pay much closer attention. If you do not adequately explain away an important point that the plaintiff's attorney made, then you could draw attention to a major weakness in your case.

The following is a line of questioning that a plaintiff's attorney might use against a doctor to make them look bad in front of a jury. It is for a case of missed cholecystitis.

Did you consider cholecystitis as a possible diagnosis in my client? *Yes.*
Did you do an ultrasound to confirm this possibility? *No.*
Can right-sided abdominal pain be evidence of cholecystitis? *Yes.*
Did the patient have right-sided abdominal pain? *Yes.*
Can you get fever in cholecystitis? *Yes.*
Did my client have a fever? *Yes.*
Can you get an increased heart rate in cholecystitis? *Yes.*
Did the patient have increased heart rate? *Yes.*
Did you call in a surgeon? *No.*
Did you admit the patient? *No.*

As you can see, if you are the doctor, this line of questioning would make you feel very uncomfortable on the stand. You realize that if you could explain the answers more thoroughly, you would not sound so bad. But in this scenario, you do not have that option.

If your attorney did his or her job properly, then it means you already addressed each and every one of these issues in his or her direct examination of you. Therefore, these answers will not pack as much of a punch, as they are after you have already explained all of your case.

If the plaintiff's attorney gets first shot at you (the usual circumstance), your attorney will in some fashion address each point the plaintiff's attorney made and allow you to explain it away. And because you had the final word, your explanation will be fresher in the jury's mind.

Cross-examination tips:
– Do not be too quick to agree with the plaintiff's attorney.
– Answer a question with a question (but do not overdo it).
– Be wary of any questions that ask you to agree with something.
– Do not parry with the attorney.
– Look at the jury when answering questions.
– Use the three-second rule and think about the question before you give your response.

Do not be too quick to agree with the plaintiff's attorney
If possible, try to find a reason to disagree with the plaintiff's attorney's statement. Especially if it is something that the attorney expects you to agree with.

For instance, if the lawyer states "morphine is a really strong medicine," say, "I can't answer that with a yes or no unless you let me explain," or simply, "No it isn't." In all likelihood, they will not let you explain. However, the assumption by plaintiff's attorney is that you will say yes to this seemingly innocuous question. When you do not answer the way they expect, this will alter their game plan and throw them off a little bit.

The allowance for a full explanation scenario
Other states allow you to "explain further." Because it is hard to restrict tricky plaintiff questions to a simple yes or no, being able to explain in detail is definitely to your advantage.

If you are allowed to give explanations, it is much easier. Repeating the above example, "morphine is a really strong medicine," you say, "No, it isn't. There are much stronger medicines than morphine available: Dilaudid, Stadol, Nubain, Fentanyl …."

So much in medicine is subjective, and if you can give a good, coherent explanation as to why the "simple proposition" is incorrect, you can disrupt the plaintiff's attorney's quick-fire line of questions. The following is the same line of questions as in the previous scenario, only now we can give explanations:

Did you consider cholecystitis as a possible diagnosis in my client? *Yes, any time a person has right-sided abdominal pain, cholecystitis is a possibility.* Did you do an ultrasound to confirm this possibility? *No, the patient had many other symptoms that made cholecystitis less likely, including normal lab values, and therefore, a right upper quadrant ultrasound was not required.* Can right-sided abdominal pain be evidence of cholecystitis? *Yes, if it is right upper quadrant pain, but my patient had right LOWER quadrant pain and a copious vaginal discharge, verified by pelvic exam.*

Did the patient have right-sided abdominal pain? *This question is no longer necessary.*

Can you get fever in cholecystits? *Yes, and dozens of other conditions.*

Did my client have a fever? *Yes, but only on arrival to the emergency department. Her temperature was normal by the time she was discharged from the hospital.*

Can you get an increased heart rate in cholecystitis? *Yes, and with dozens of other medical conditions.*

Did the patient have increased heart rate? *Yes on arrival, but it was normal after I fully hydrated her with two liters of normal saline.*

Did you call in a surgeon? *No, in this case of a patient with pelvic inflammatory disease, a surgeon is not an appropriate consult.*

Did you admit the patient? *No, the patient did not meet criteria for admission.*

As you can see, living in a state that allows you to give explanations with your answer is a huge advantage. You can do damage control as you are giving your answer, not preventatively, and not after the fact as in the prior scenario.

If a window opens up with an open-ended question, spout a quick coherent version of your defense.

Some attorneys will cut you off before you can finish your explanation (often making them look rude). Others will let you continue on as long as you speak. Just make sure that whatever you say is helpful. Remember, "Do no harm" applies to your testimony as well.

Other cross-examination tips
Answer a question with a question
The best way to upset an examiner, and the one thing that the questioner never wants to hear from a witness, is a question from the witness. Find a portion of the question asked that you find vague or too general and ask him a question. If the attorneys avoid your question, they look bad and evasive. Do not overdo this or else you will appear obstructive. If the question is harmless, and not a key issue in the case, give a simple answer.

Be ready to summarize your whole case in a few quick sentences
On rare occasions, the cross-examining attorney will ask you to elaborate on an issue. This is your opening to talk and keep talking about that question and your entire defense.

How do you know when to spew your defense? Your attorney will prepare you and will teach you what phrases are triggers for you. Each case is different, but as an example, if you have a case where the defendants acted in a conservative manner and the patient eventually required surgery, the buzz word would be conservative. Any chance the defendants get, they want to spit out that they acted in a deliberate conservative manner, rather than just doing surgery for surgery's sake. Then, waiting for an opening, such as "why did you proceed the way you did," the defendants open both barrels and declare their prepared defense statement.

Be wary of any questions that ask whether you agree with something
For instance,

Q: Do you agree or disagree with this statement?

These situations are designed to trap you. Often, this innocent sounding question deals with critical facts in your case. It is structured in such a way that you usually want to agree with the statement. However, if you do, it will be twisted around to make you look bad.

Your goal in this case is to find an intelligent way to disagree with the statement. If it is a quote from an article or book, ask what year that article was sourced from. Chances are high that the article is old enough for you to disagree with their statement as being "out of date."

It is critically important that you completely understand what you are agreeing/disagreeing with. Therefore, before giving any opinions, you must ask, "Can I see the context of where you are getting that statement?" This is both for your own edification and as a stall tactic to give you more time to configure a good response.

Stay cool at all times
Do not lose your control. Do not appear angry. Do not appear frustrated. In fact, try to present a calm emotionless façade. Even if you are being hammered by the attorneys who could even yell at you (yes, some attorneys do this for dramatic effect to rattle you), you must continue to remain controlled. If they can disrupt your demeanor, it will harm your case.

Do not parry with the attorney
They do this for a living. You will lose the battle and may also look really bad in process.

Look at the jury when answering questions
Eye contact goes a long way when trying to connect with a juror. However, if it makes you uncomfortable to look directly at the jurors, then at least look in their direction.

Never sound condescending, even when the attorney has just insulted you

Your tone of voice is critical. Imagine how the phrase "sure you can" sounds with both a straightforward or sarcastic delivery. It makes all the difference between winning and losing. If the jurors think you are condescending or sarcastic, they will want to find fault against you. If they like you, they are more inclined to believe you.

My father has recounted to me dozens of cases where physicians who had not committed malpractice had some degree of fault assigned to them by the jury simply because their "attitude" induced the jurors to want to punish them. It should not be this way as the facts should be the sole basis on which to make a decision of fault. However, the truth is that if jurors do not like you, they will hurt you; particularly, if there is a very sympathetic plaintiff.

Do not be fooled by the plaintiff's attorney

Use the "three-second" rule when answering questions. In other words, always take a little bit of time to carefully consider your answer. In this regard, remember some advice from the deposition, *beware of double negative questions.*

For instance,

Q: Did you not leave the scissor inside of Mr. Plaintiff?

If you answer with a simple "yes," you are really saying, "yes, I did not leave the scissor inside …," which actually means "no," not "yes." To this type of confusing question, your answer should be

A: I do not understand your question.

or

A: I cannot answer yes or no the way you have phrased it.

Do not answer something you do not understand

This sounds simple, but as in the deposition, if you are not 100% sure of what is being asked, do not answer it. Say, "I don't understand the question as asked." Do not allow the attorney to get away with his or her attempts to confuse you.

Beware of anything given to you by plaintiff's attorney to look at on the stand

Assume that anything the plaintiff's attorney gives you to look at on the stand is there to harm you. Even if a diagram looks harmless, chances are there is something that is taken out of context. Be very careful before agreeing with the attorney regarding anything on that diagram.

Take time to carefully review every single word and diagram on that paper. Do not allow yourself to be rushed. The jury will appreciate a doctor who is careful and cautious.

> Go beyond the three-second rule when looking at something handed to you by the plaintiff's attorney while you are on the stand. The attorney is counting on the fact that you will rush and miss something.

Use layman's terms at all times when answering questions

Obviously, you will have to use medical terminology. You should use medical terms to a certain degree. However, medical jargon can be difficult for jurors to understand. If you must use a medical term, follow it up with a layman's explanation of it.

Your goal here, unlike the deposition, is to make your language as clear and easy as possible for the jury to understand. Many plaintiff's experts try to earn their money by peppering their explanations with fancy medical mumbo jumbo. It makes them sound important. It also can make them unintelligible to the jury.

If the jurors understand you, but not the plaintiff's expert, they are more likely to find for the defense. Also, if you can be the one to teach the jury the medical information, it will go a long way toward strengthening your defense.

Make sure you know your deposition verbatim

Chances are, at some point in the plaintiff's attorneys' examination of you, they will pull out your deposition to confront you with something you said. They may attempt to contradict your testimony. Make sure you know it well enough to refute them with nearby lines that put everything in its proper context. Below is a line of questioning from a state where you are allowed to give further explanation.

Q: Is it true that part of the standard of care of medicine is good charting?
A: Yes.

Q: Is it also true that your chart (which the plaintiff's attorney has blown up to a five foot size demonstration piece) is incomplete?
A: No. The information is there.

Attorney is stunned with this unexpected answer and immediately pulls out a copy of the deposition.

Q: Doctor, please read back to me page 55 line 4.
   (This is where you should quickly read page 54, page 55, and page 56 to
   yourself before reading anything out loud)
A: "Question: You did not on the front page, as you've already alluded to,
   make any entries regarding time course, quality, location associated
   with severity, exacerbation or relief on that left-hand column, correct?
   Answer: Yes, like …"

   Plaintiff's attorney interrupts.

Q: So you have changed your testimony doctor? Clearly, you said in your
   deposition that you did not have a completed chart. How can you say to
   this jury that you did?
A: Well, if you look about 10 lines prior to what you just asked me to read,
   line 15 on the previous page, you will see "would you read that for me
   please." You asked me in the deposition to read my chart for you and
   then asked me if there were spaces that I did not fill out. Therefore,
   although certain spaces on the front page were left empty, the information is in the chart; just not in those spaces you just made me read about.
   If you will allow me a moment, I will be happy to show you on my chart
   where all of that information is located.

   Plaintiff gives up and moves to another topic.
   Lesson learned here: Whoever knows the deposition better scores more
points. If you were not careful and had not taken the time to read the context of the quote you were being asked to recite, you would have fallen for
the plaintiff's trick and appeared to be changing your testimony. Instead, it
made the plaintiff look foolish, like he was taking things out of context. And
the last thing he or she wanted was for you to SHOW him or her that your
chart was actually complete.
   If you had not known your deposition well, you might also have been
caught unaware of your statements and that surprise you feel in being trapped
by the plaintiff could be perceived by the jury as being caught in a lie.
   Knowing your deposition well protects you from any surprises. You know
exactly what is in there, good and bad, and you know what the plaintiff's
attorney will likely use against you. Therefore, you can never be confronted
with testimony you do not remember. And you can retort with complete
confidence.
   Also, there is a good chance that the plaintiff's attorneys simply picked
out parts of your deposition that they feel could best be used against you.
They likely do not have it all memorized. Therefore, they may not be able to
counter your attack.

In this example, had the plaintiff's attorney known the deposition better, he or she could have said, "in that particular section, I asked you to read, but on page so and so, line x (which he reads) I simply asked you if there were sections of the chart left incomplete, and you said yes. Are you refuting that answer now?"

You still have the opportunity to say, "the spaces were incomplete in that section, but the information was present elsewhere." But at least the plaintiff's attorney would have got a jab in and not looked so foolish. By not knowing the deposition well enough, he or she was the one who got caught, not you.

Do not lie!

Rest assured, if you change your testimony from your deposition, it will be used against you. However, if you noticed a way to salvage a poor deposition answer with a clarification, be prepared to give your better answer in a convincing manner. You will be challenged on it, and you will need to defend yourself in a way that makes you look confident but not arrogant.

Do not fidget

Keep your hands at your lap when you are testifying. If you need to wear glasses during your testimony, then wear them at all times. To put them on and then take them off after each question is annoying and distracting.

Even when you are not testifying but are in court, you will be under scrutiny by the jury. You must not comment, facially or through body language, your approval or disapproval of any witnesses' testimony. Do not take notes or write notes to your attorney in front of the jury. If you must, wait until a break in the action. The reason is that if you write notes, the jury will see it and wonder if what was going on was damaging to your case.

You might call attention to something bad that the jury would have ignored otherwise. Also, some jurors take offense to your expressions of disapproval, especially with the plaintiff on the stand.

After the plaintiff's attorney rests

When the plaintiff's attorneys finish presenting their part of the case, they rest. At this point, there is an opening for you, the defendant, to get out of the case.

Your attorney can make a *motion to dismiss the complaint* (This verbal motion is a request to the court). The basis of this being that the plaintiff has not proven his or her case. Although it is not common, a judge can rule at that point to dismiss the case. Or in the situation with multiple defendants, certain defendants could be dismissed from the case at this time.

Defendant begins the case

It may seem unfair that the plaintiff gets the first shot at you, even before your own attorney. This is not how it appears on television. If the plaintiff's attorneys decide for some reason not to call you in their case, your attorney will get to question you first; a big advantage.

What is so great about your attorney's direct examination of you? It is easy. Low stress. You get to say everything about your case that the plaintiff's attorney left out. You get to teach the jury certain aspects of medicine. If you can be a convincing teacher, then you will become the best and most important witness/expert at trial. And jurors who learn from you are likely to believe your point of view. They are more likely to find for the defense.

In addition, you will get an opportunity to show your personality, your intelligence, and, most importantly, that your treatment was in conformity with good and accepted medical practice. The negative aspect of this part of your case is that, for jurors, it is also pretty boring. They know that your attorney is only going to ask you questions that make you sound good. Therefore, it is a skilled attorney that can keep the jury awake and expose all the flaws in the plaintiff's case.

> Use the examination by your attorney as an opportunity to teach the jury, not just defend your case. You are an expert too.

After the defense rests, but before the verdict

There is another opportunity to have your case dismissed. Your attorney can, at this time, make a verbal *motion for a directed verdict*. A directed verdict is when a judge will make the ruling as to who wins.

It is an unusual situation if this does occur, but sometimes, the case is very one-sided, supporting the defense. As an example, the defense attorney may have skewered the plaintiff's experts and got them to agree with the defense's case. Or made it clear that the expert was lying. In this situation, the defense attorney will state that the plaintiff has not sustained a departure (i.e., departure from good and accepted medical practice, which is a proximate cause of the plaintiff's injuries) because any apparent departures were refuted by both plaintiff's experts and defense's experts. If there are no departures, there is no case, and the judge should rule for the defendant.

The judge is not required to accept the motion or deny it at that time (although it is most commonly denied). He or she has a third choice: reserve judgment until after the verdict is in. Of course, the point is pretty much moot if the defendant wins.

However, if the judge reserves judgment, and the verdict is for the plaintiff, the judge could at this time accept the motion and direct the verdict for the defendant. This is a highly unusual scenario that almost never occurs. Nevertheless, it is still possible, and it is your attorney's job to keep any avenue of winning available to you if the situation warrants it.

Closing statements (summation)

This ties the whole case together. Trials are rarely won or lost by this time as the jurors have usually made up their minds by now. However, a skilled attorney can manipulate the facts and present them in such a way that jurors might look more at certain facts than others when they go to deliberate.

The rules on what can be included in the closing statements are usually pretty lax. You cannot introduce a new concept not brought up in trial. Otherwise, your only limitations are the time allotted by the judge.

Jury charges

The judge must "charge" the jury with the law. What does this mean? Both sides must present their "requests to charge" to the judge to rule as to which points of law the jury must follow to decide the verdict. A skilled attorney can try to convince the judge to accept his or her requests to charge. This can go a long way to winning or losing.

Seriously. Why? There are proposed charges that are submitted by both sides, the wording of which can help you win your case even if the jury found some errors on your part. For instance, if the judge charges that liability is found if there is a *preponderance of evidence* against the defendant, it means that there is just enough evidence to make it more likely than not that the fact the plaintiff is seeking is true. It is the lowest standard and easier to prove and thus is more advantageous to the plaintiff.

However, there is another standard that could be used, depending on the state's laws and what the judge will accept, called *clear and convincing evidence*, which requires a high degree of certainty that the assertion against the defendant is true. This is much more difficult to prove and is beneficial to the defendant. The *beyond a reasonable doubt* is the most strict standard, but it is used only in criminal cases.

Jury deliberation

When the jurors leave the courtroom to deliberate, that is, confer formally to reach a decision on the case, there is not much left for you to do. For the most part, you just wait for their determination, which could take an hour, several hours, or possibly several days. However, depending on how the attorneys perceive the outcome of the trial, there could be a last minute settlement. The longer jury deliberation lasts, as a general rule, the more it favors the plaintiff (because it is assumed that what is taking a long time is the calculation of damages, which does not occur in a defendant's verdict).

If something like this happens, and in particular if you have a high-damages case, your insurance company will be fearful that the jury is deciding on how many zeros to award to the plaintiff and will want to get out for a lower cost. Sometimes juries write a note to the judge asking for more evidence, clarifications, or even a calculator! Thus, if the jury is asking peculiar questions and spending a long time deciding the case, your insurer may opt for a last minute settlement. If you have the *consent to settle* clause in your policy, they cannot force you to settle, but they may try to apply pressure to you to give consent. If you do not have this clause in your policy, you will have no choice.

To render a verdict, in most civil cases, more than a majority of jurors is generally needed. How many jurors are needed to have a verdict varies widely. Usually, only criminal cases require a unanimous verdict. If enough jurors cannot come to an agreement, they cannot deliver a verdict, and thus it creates a situation called a *hung jury*. If this happens, there will need to be a whole new trial with a brand new jury.

Juror actions can also lead to a mistrial—an invalid trial caused by fundamental error that requires a whole new trial. Sometimes jurors violate the jury code of conduct, such as discussing the case with one another before deliberation, talking with plaintiffs or defendants, and using extraneous information to help make their judgment. Although it is rare, on occasion, a juror may use the Internet or local library to do some extra research on the case. However, this is not permitted as the jurors are supposed to use only the facts as discussed in the trial. Thus, if this behavior is discovered, a mistrial can be declared.

Damages

If the jurors decide for the plaintiff, the topic of damages—assigning a monetary value to the injury incurred—will be discussed. In doing so, they will have two separate categories to address: economic and noneconomic damages.

Economic damages provide compensation for objectively verifiable monetary losses such as past and future medical expenses and loss of past and future earnings. When making the determination of medical expenses, sometimes collateral sources are not taken into consideration. For instance, patients who are on Medicaid, and do not pay their bill, can still ask the jury to award damages for the medical expenses they did not pay. As a result, many states have reformed this practice (see Appendix C for the list of states that allow jurors to assess collateral sources). Many jurors, after trial, find out that they awarded millions of dollars to a patient on the basis of their immense hospital bill, only to find out that the patient never paid the bill anyway, and are infuriated at the system that deliberately kept them ignorant of those facts. Thus, this statute has huge implications on the final verdict amount.

Noneconomic damages are subjective and hard to measure. Examples of these are pain and suffering, inconvenience, emotional distress, loss of consortium (intercourse with spouse), and loss of enjoyment of life. Many states have capped these nonquantifiable damages to help rein in exorbitant jury awards.

> When you hear about tort reform caps on pain and suffering, they are referring to noneconomic damages only.

There is a third category: *punitive damages*. These are only awarded to inflict an economic punishment on defendants who the jury feels have acted recklessly or maliciously. These are considered a separate category because they are not compensatory.

The verdict

Hopefully, you will get a defendant's verdict. And if you are in court for the verdict, and win, be professional and accept your victory with dignity. After all, the case is not technically over until the plaintiff's attorney exhausts all appeals. And that could be another multistep process, taking a year or longer if the plaintiff's attorney pursues it. This course of action is explained in detail in Chapter 10.

Chapter 10 **What to do if you lose?**

Once you hear that the verdict is for the plaintiff, you will likely not hear anything else. Although you may have just lost your case, this does not necessarily mean that this is the end. There is a lot that can go on behind the scenes.

> Although losing your case can be the end of the road, it can actually be the beginning of a new road leading to a new trial.

Depending on the details of your trial, there may be grounds for an appeal. Appeals to a higher court, if accepted, can lead to a number of scenarios:
1 a new trial
2 a reduction in damages
3 affirmance or reversal of the lower court's decision

What are the steps to get an appeal?

Before your lawyer leaves the courtroom, after the verdict, there are some things that will happen.

Your attorney will propose some postverdict motions to the judge in an effort to get the same result as if you had an instant appeal.

It is possible that in your case there was such a flagrant disregard of the evidence by the jury that the judge will immediately overturn the verdict and hand it to you, the defendant.

Why would the judge do this? There was no basis for the verdict by the credible evidence but the jury felt sympathy for the plaintiff, and/or hated the defendant, or got sidetracked by minor issues.

How to Survive a Medical Malpractice Lawsuit. By © Ilene R. Brenner. Published 2010 Blackwell Publishing.

To win this, your attorney would have to show that there was no valid line of reasoning and permissible inference that could possibly lead rational people to the conclusion reached by the jury on the evidence presented at trial. In other words, the verdict was utterly irrational.

To obtain this result, your attorney would make a *motion for a directed verdict.*

Most of the motions are performed with the intent of establishing grounds for appeal. However, there is always a small chance that there would be a ruling for you (very small, and unlikely, but there nevertheless).

As an example of trial court error, let us say it is 4:30 pm and the defense attorney is cross-examining the plaintiff's expert. To wrap up for the day, the judge could insist that you have five questions or five minutes to finish up, which ever happens first. And the judge could stipulate that whether you like it or not, you are done; that witness will not return the next day.

You would be surprised by the bizarre abuses of power judges wield. These abuses can be used as a basis for a new trial. All these motions can be denied or reserved from the bench. I explained in the previous chapter that the judge can rule immediately or reserve judgment. These motions, however, can sometimes sit on a judge's desk for months.

After the motions, typically the losing party is the one who will order an abstract of the trial record, in some jurisdictions called "clerks minutes," which is essential to obtain a *judgment* (see the following text for details on judgments).

Within the next week or two, the losing party will enter a judgment with the clerk of the court. This is defined as a final disposition of the case. In layman's terms, it is an official filing of the verdict. This is necessary because the loser can appeal from the judgment, and the winner (if the plaintiff) can pursue collection of the monetary award at this point.

Your attorney will then file a notice of appeal. This is exactly the way it sounds; they are notifying the appellate court that an appeal is imminent. However, it takes months to perfect the appeal.

The insurance company issues a bond to protect the plaintiff's judgment (e.g., money they were awarded from the trial) so that if the defendant loses the appeal, the plaintiff gets the judgment plus interest.

How can I get my attorney to file for an appeal?

Your attorney will file an appeal at the insurance company's behest. What they will take into consideration are the chances of winning the appeal, versus the cost of the appeal, and the amount of the verdict.

This is the case even if you have *consent to settle* in your policy. Once a judgment has been entered, all consent rights end. Oftentimes, if there is a very large verdict (excessive), the insurance company will try to cut a deal with the plaintiff: "If you reduce the twenty million dollar judgment down to the policy limits, then we will terminate the appeal process."

> Even if you have *consent to settle* in your policy, you have very little say in whether your case gets appealed.

If the insurance company can settle the judgment, it is a win-win for both parties: the insurance covers the policy limits without overage to the doctor. Also for the plaintiff, though winning the appeal is still achievable, there is still the possibility of losing the second trial without grounds to appeal. The insurance company after the second trial could have spent twice as much money for the same or worse result (the new jury could come in with a larger monetary verdict).

Why would the plaintiff give up most of their verdict? The prospect of a certain, immediate payment versus a larger uncertain payment makes a settlement very attractive. The plaintiff's attorney gets the immediate use of his fee, and the plaintiff gets the immediate use of the balance of the settlement. Also, it prevents the appellate division from declaring the verdict too excessive and ordering a new trial on damages.

> Insurance companies often settle cases that could go for an appeal to negotiate a lower payment than the verdict.

They can, and will, do this without any input from you.

You can ask, implore, and encourage your attorney to pursue an appeal. However, it is left to the insurance company's discretion, and they may refuse your insistence to appeal. A simple appeal can be costly, from $15,000 to $25,000.

> Appeals are complicated and involve months of work to prepare.

In fact, once you get to a judgment, your attorney–client relationship may or may not end depending on the jurisdiction. Even if you are allowed to pursue an appeal, the insurance company may opt to transfer your case to another law firm, typically an appellate specialist. Again, although you like and trust your attorney, you have no choice.

Many doctors, at this point, would probably rather want the case to just end. It has been over 2–3 years of their life at this point, and they would rather let it end now in a loss than prolong the process further. Winning an appeal usually means getting a new trial and all of the stress factors that go along with it.

No matter how much we try to convince ourselves that this is just a game, and no matter how well we played the game, the fact is we are not just faceless physicians. We are people who fear losing our livelihood, our self-respect, our reputation, and our compassion. Obviously, the process of a lawsuit is a long and painful journey. Physicians would do just about anything to prevent one; hence, the widespread problem of defensive medicine. The next chapters begin Section 2, which describes many different ways to decrease the likelihood of being sued.

Section 2 An ounce of prevention

Chapter 11 **Why doctors get sued**

Now that you have read everything about the lawsuit process, wouldn't it be great to prevent getting sued in the first place?

There are many people who tout ways to prevent a lawsuit. There are scores of books and courses dedicated to this topic. But the truth is nothing can completely prevent a lawsuit. Although there are some things that can be done to decrease the likelihood of getting sued, statistically, most doctors will get sued at least once during their career. This section includes some preventative tips and advice that will set you up to have a more easily defended lawsuit.

What can be done to prevent getting sued?

To answer that you need to find out why people sue doctors. Generally, patients become plaintiffs when two conditions are met: (1) patients have something go wrong with their medical care and (2) patients and/or their families are angry.

Bad outcome

As medicine is not an exact science, there is a likelihood that even if an excellent medical care is given, an adverse outcome might result. If a surgeon explains that a surgery is 95% successful, then that means statistically 5% will be unsuccessful. Five percent equates to 5 of every 100 patients. Think about how many patients you see and do the math yourself. Clearly, the statistics alone will create millions of patients with bad outcomes.

> Statistically every physician will have a patient who suffers a bad outcome. It does not mean you are a bad doctor. It does not mean you are negligent.

How to Survive a Medical Malpractice Lawsuit. By © Ilene R. Brenner. Published 2010 Blackwell Publishing.

Some doctors have patients with worse outcomes than others. Some surgeons have patients with more post-op infections than others. Some doctors have more cases needing peer review than others. If you fall into this category, then you need to do something to attempt to improve upon your care. However, getting given physicians to admit that they need to accept some blame for their patient's bad outcome is a difficult proposition.

> If you have greater than average numbers of patients with bad outcomes, you may want to do a chart review to see whether there is room for improvement or simply bad luck.

But if you are reading this book, then you are a physician who is interested in championing your own defense. And thus, you should do what you can to decrease the likelihood of a bad outcome. And that means keeping up with evidence-based medicine (EBM) and CMEs (Continuing Medical Education). It means treating every bad outcome as a learning experience. "Can I prevent a similar occurrence in the future?" is the question you should be asking yourself.

Also, avoid drinking alcohol or taking certain medications the day that you work (or even the night before if the drug's half-life is such that it still has effects 8 hours after discontinuance). If you would recommend not taking a medicine while driving or using heavy machinery, you should also not take it before or while working.

Using vehicular manslaughter as an analogy, if you are sober and cause a car accident that kills someone, it is called an accident. If you are above the legal limit for alcohol consumption in the same instance, you go to jail for manslaughter. The same thing is true with medical malpractice. If something goes wrong with a patient, you can call it a bad outcome. If you had alcohol or medicine on board that could theoretically make you impaired (even if it did not), your bad outcome becomes malpractice and you will likely have to settle out of the case if that information is allowed to be told to a jury as evidence at trial.

If something goes wrong, should I apologize?

This is a very hard to answer question. Multiple studies have shown that apologizing to patients when something goes wrong with the patient's care can help prevent a lawsuit. Patients appreciate when a doctor feels remorse and often that is the deciding factor when not suing.

However, in many states, your apology is not protected under the law and can be used against you in court as an *Admission Against Interest*. Other states protect your apology just as peer review is protected (see Appendix D for the specific states' details).

If your apology is not protected, you are in a tricky situation. On the one hand, apologizing can help prevent a lawsuit. On the other hand, if sued, you are much more likely to lose the case because you admitted guilt.

> Angry patient + bad outcome = medical malpractice lawsuit. You cannot control bad outcome so do what you can to have less angry patients.

Angry patients

What makes patients angry?

1 Doctors who act like they do not care about their patients' welfare.
2 Doctors who do not listen to their patients' (and their families') concerns.
3 Doctors who are rude to their patients.
4 Doctors who are sarcastic to their patients.
5 Doctors who are unavailable to their patients.
6 Doctors who condescend to the patients.
7 Doctors who do not spend any time with the patient.
8 Doctors who cancel patients' appointments.
9 Doctors who have exceedingly long wait times to get an appointment and long wait times in the waiting room.
10 Constantly being relegated to see the physician extender instead of the physician.
11 Being told by another doctor that bad care was given to them.
12 Receiving a bill for care that was a bad outcome. In the same vein, patients also get angry when they get huge bills for an incorrect diagnosis. Some patients get angry when they get a large bill for the numerous tests that were performed simply to find nothing significantly wrong.

What can you do to prevent your patients from being angry with you?

1 Show interest, care, and concern. You may be the most caring doctor on the planet, but if you do not communicate that to your patient, it will not matter. To that end, there are some things that you can do to create the aura of a caring, concerned doctor:

   a) *Sit down* when talking with your patients. Studies show that patients perceive the amount of time the doctor spends with the patient as much longer if a doctor is seated instead of standing (Strasser and Palmer, 2005).

   b) *Use eye contact.* A doctor with their head buried in their chart gives the appearance of someone who is not listening.

c) *Nod*. An occasional nod to the patient tells them you are paying attention to what they are saying.

d) *Let the patient speak*. Obviously, a patient who talks too much can waste most valuable time. However, much of the reason patients seek the services of a physician is to achieve some kind of validation for their suffering. They want to know that there is someone who will listen to their concerns. Patients are paying you to be that someone.

e) *Use the patient's words*. If you use some of the patients' own words when speaking to them, they will know you were paying attention to them.

> Patients prefer physicians to sit rather than stand when taking a history. Patients perceive these physicians as being more compassionate.

2 Leave your attitude at the door.

You may have just spent the past hour fruitlessly arguing with the insurance company for a preauthorization. You may be getting a divorce. Your kids may all be going to college at once. You may not be sleeping because of a new baby. You may be pregnant. Your wife may be pregnant. You may be getting audited.

It does not matter what kind of travesty is occurring in your life. You need to let that go when seeing patients. If you are upset and annoyed, chances are you will communicate that to your patients, and they will become upset and annoyed.

3 Try to be available to your patients.

I know that you work too hard for too little money, and it does not seem worth it to spend too much time dealing with patient concerns outside of office hours. However, doctors who are not available to their patients are viewed as uncaring.

With modern technology, there are many ways to connect with patients. You could set up an email system of communication in addition to your usual answering service.

Regarding your answering service, call it yourself from time to time. See what they are like. Do you receive a page from them promptly? If a patient calls the answering service and the service does not page you, the patient thinks you got the page and ignored them. Ensuring that your paging service functions properly can go a long way to keep your patients satisfied.

Another strategy of better communication is using a physician extender as a bridge (see Chapter 14 for more information on physician extender liability issues). They can field calls and screen out the ones who absolutely must talk with you. They can also call patients with results from tests that were performed. Patients who get prompt results of their lab tests tend to be happier. Plus, it prevents little things like radiology over-reads which show masses, from falling through the cracks. Missed cancer diagnoses from tests performed but not reported to patients is a common reason for lawsuits.

Patients are happy when they feel connected and can connect with their physician. Use available technology to aid you.

4 Do not ever speak in a condescending manner to your patients.

When patients come to you, it is because they trust you, the doctor, to help them become well. Although their questions may be mundane and annoying at times, speaking to them in a way that demeans them or makes them feel stupid for even asking the question is wrong for many reasons.

For one, it destroys the foundation of trust between doctor and patient, which is so important in the healing process. For another, it makes the patient upset and primed to find something you did wrong to make you feel stupid. It may make them seek revenge in the form of a lawsuit.

Treat your patients with respect.

5 Spend sufficient time with each patient.

There is nothing worse than a patient encounter where the patient feels rushed. As mentioned earlier, sit down whenever possible. Do not look at your watch. And if called out of the room, ensure to come back before finishing up. Even if someone else can finish up for you, at least pop in for a brief second. That way the patient will not feel so abandoned.

Clearly in this era of decreased reimbursement, it is necessary for a viable practice to see at least four patients per hour. Certainly, this does not leave much time for patient care. However, do your best to make the patients feel like they got some value for their time.

Sometimes patients merely want validation for their problems. Use verbal and nonverbal cues to indicate you are listening to their complaint.

6 If you cancel a patient's appointment, ensure it is rescheduled within a reasonable period of time.

Stuff happens. Sometimes your schedule needs to be cleared after appointments are made. Ensure your staff goes the extra mile to contact every person affected and make them a priority to see you the moment you become available.

Ensure the patient is informed as early as possible of an appointment cancellation. If the patient shows up for a cancelled appointment, it will make them very upset.

7 Patients should be able to get an appointment with you within a reasonable period of time.

Most physicians have a protocol for patients to get in: VIPs get in immediately, patients seen in the emergency department within 1 or 2 days, patients with urgent complaints within a few days, patients with checkups within a few weeks, and self-pay patients within a few designated slots per month.

Although this system is not completely unreasonable, it is usually patient driven, meaning a patient must insist or else they will not get a prompt appointment. All too often, patients simply call and ask for an appointment, and medical staffs do not prod them with questions that would get them an appointment within the prescribed period of time.

Patients get angry when they are forced to go to the emergency department, and wait there for hours, for a nonemergency that could have been seen in your office *if* you had actually given them an appointment in a reasonable period of time.

8 Patients should not have to wait 2 hours in a doctor's office waiting room for their scheduled appointment.

Obviously, there are many factors that could cause a doctor's schedule to be very delayed. However, in this era of cell phones that do text messaging and instant email, there is an opportunity to inform patients of a long delay.

As your Garmin gives you helpful traffic updates that give estimated delay times, imagine how happy your patients would be to get a message informing them of your delay.

The message in this section is not that we all have to be technological geniuses to keep our patients happy. However, paying attention to inefficiencies that cause long wait times, and finding ways of communicating with your patients to let them know that their valuable time was not unnecessarily wasted in the waiting room, goes a long way to keeping your patients happy. And happy patients rarely sue doctors.

9 Make the long wait in the waiting room of the emergency department more bearable.

There are some proven methods of increasing patient satisfaction:

a) greeters

b) easily available food

    c) television

    d) comfortable seating

    e) tolerable noise level

10 Patients presenting to your office expect to see you. Use your physician extenders to support you, not supplant you.

Although most patients do not mind seeing a physician extender from time to time, most patients are there to see you, the medical doctor. And they pay to see you. Many patients feel that paying to see you but seeing a physician extender instead is a "bait and switch."

If you do not see the patients yourself, you will eventually alienate your patients. Alienated patients are more likely to sue if something goes wrong. What is the solution? You could ensure that any patient who saw a physician extender on this visit will definitely see the doctor on the next visit.

You could also create a system where you ensure that even if a patient sees a physician extender, they still get to see you to ask a few questions if need be. I am not suggesting these are all great solutions and the only solutions available. However, it is my attempt to think outside of the box; to come up with ways to mitigate the frustration that patients feel when seeing a physician extender in place of the physician.

11 Never criticize another doctor's care in front of the patient. Never make disparaging comments about another doctor's care in the medical record.

You may be surprised to hear this, but a large number of plaintiffs admit that they decided to sue when their doctor told them that another doctor's care was less than adequate. In addition, a large number of patients who are angry and thinking about suing will review the medical record looking for a reason. If you place an inappropriate comment regarding another doctor's care in that record, it will likely trigger a lawsuit.

Why should you care if something you say or write leads to another doctor being sued? For one, it is unprofessional. There is a time and place to criticize another doctor. There are protocols for this occurrence: every hospital has a quality assurance/risk management/peer review system. If you do not approve of how a physician handled a patient of yours, then send it through peer review. Many patients' charts end up in peer review because of the value of hindsight as a chief source of criticism. But just because your patient ended up sicker after seeing a physician, it does not mean malpractice occurred.

If you say or write something that implicates another doctor, then you become judge and jury regarding this doctor's medical treatment. Yet every doctor is entitled to peer review; something you just denied them.

Second, your actions can get you pulled into the lawsuit yourself. Do not think you are automatically exempt from being sued yourself. Loyal patients will become disloyal when their attorney convinces them that it is best to sue everybody involved, which includes you.

This does not contradict earlier advice regarding thorough documentation. If you have a disagreement regarding patient care, try not to use judgmental and inflammatory language. Just state the facts. For instance, "I called Dr. Y at 3:10 am to get a surgical evaluation. Dr. Y returned my call at 3:50 am and felt that this patient did not warrant admission. I then spoke with the hospitalist Dr. Z, who agreed to admit the patient." You do need to protect yourself, but do not go out of your way to implicate another physician.

> A large number of patients sue their doctor because other doctors told them there was malpractice.

12 In general, with the high cost of medicine and poor coverage by insurance, patients are dismayed to receive large bills that they are responsible for paying. This frustration is further compounded when they or their relative have a bad outcome. After all, why should they spend money on care that did not help?

What should a physician do in this case? Certainly, if no malpractice was committed, the physician should feel justified to collect payment for services that were rendered. Once the poor outcome has occurred, the physician must weigh too the pros and cons of seeking collection of those funds. It may prevent a lawsuit if you waive the fee. Although you may deserve payment as there was no malpractice, the reality is that preventing a lawsuit likely is worth the loss of a fee on this particular patient.

Also, you need to be careful about bills that are aggressively pursued by collections. If you try to collect every dime from every patient, you will likely have an increase in lawsuits. One way of assuaging this problem is through good, clear communication with both the patients and their family before a treatment plan or procedure (see the Chapter 12 on *Communication Issues* for more information). If the family is aware of the true risks and likelihood of a poor outcome (e.g., patient is obese and smokes), then they will be more tolerant of the eventual receipt of a bill for services.

Sometimes a person's disease condition does not immediately reveal itself. You can present to the emergency department with symptoms one day, get a whole host of negative tests, and return a day later with worsened symptoms and the same tests are now positive. Sometimes you appear to have cholecystitis and a negative ultrasound one day, and the next day end up diagnosed with a small bowel obstruction. From a physician's perspective, this is simply part of the "art" of imprecise medical diagnosis. From a patient's perspective, it is a double bill for one diagnosis. In this situation, it may be wise to "write off" the first bill, even though there was no fault on the physician's part.

Finally, patients sometimes get upset when you do many expensive tests to rule out severe diseases such as heart attacks, only to find something relatively minor such as heartburn. In this case, I would not write off the bill. This is a situation where further communication with the patient would be of value. One physician whom I know explained to a patient in this circumstance, "Had they had a heart attack the same tests would need to be performed. As there is no way to predict who will have a heart attack prior to doing the tests, some patients will require tests and be normal." Again, communication of this before performing the tests is more effective than afterwards. See the Chapter 12 for more helpful information for better communication with your patient.

Reference

Strasser F, Palmer JL. Impact of physician sitting versus standing during patient oncology consultations. *J Pain Symptom Manage* 2005;29(5):489–97.

Chapter 12 **Communication issues**

Effective communication is essential

One day, in the Emergency Department, I had a teenage patient with an infection. After her history and examination, I wrote up the discharge paperwork and gave it to the nurse for discharge. Before the nurse came in, I spent a few minutes explaining the diagnosis and treatment plan, to both the patient and the mother. I answered numerous questions and felt I spent longer than usual in discussions for a very minor infection.

Ten minutes later, to my horror, the Nurse Manager came to me detailing a complaint about me. Apparently, the mother of the girl with whom I had just spent time giving very detailed discharge instructions claimed I told them nothing and demanded an apology. I was dumbfounded and frustrated. However, I went in there and gave the instructions again.

I could not believe that the patient's mother not only did not pay attention to a word I said, but she also made a formal complaint! I decided that although I did nothing specifically wrong, I recognized that I failed to communicate properly.

When people are under stress, they often do not think clearly. Health problems are very stressful for most people. Oftentimes, patients will ask questions, but not process the answers. They will appear as though they are paying attention and understanding what you are talking about, but in reality they did not hear anything you just told them.

> It is not what you say, it is what the patient hears.

Physicians have enough to do without having to repeat themselves multiple times. Even with redundancy in instructions, patients fail to pay attention.

How to Survive a Medical Malpractice Lawsuit. By © Ilene R. Brenner. Published 2010 Blackwell Publishing, ISBN: 978-1-4443-3130-1.

For instance, you may give your verbal instructions, the nurse will give their instructions, the patient will receive written instructions, and the patient still will not understand. Obviously, you cannot do much in these circumstances.

However, there are some strategies to improve the likelihood your patients will understand you. Drawing pictures can help explain the diagnosis better than words. Asking your patients to repeat back to you what they believe you just told them is effective. Also, having a friend or relative present who will also hear your instructions will increase the likelihood that the patients will eventually understand what they need to do.

It is imperative you do your best to communicate effectively with your patients. Besides being good for your patients' well-being, it also decreases your likelihood of being sued.

> If the patients do not understand what the doctor told them, it is a failure of communication.

Special issues with patients who speak a foreign language

We live in a multicultural society, and as such, it is likely you will face a situation where your patients do not speak English. Poor understanding of your patient during your history-taking is not an excuse for malpractice. It is in your best interest to obtain translation if needed.

If you happen to speak a foreign language, you must be fluent enough to obtain an accurate history and explain procedures, diagnoses, and treatment plans. Some physicians are partially fluent and can obtain a medical history and procedures but cannot understand questions and more complicated issues such as treatment plans. In this case, you should not "wing it." You must obtain translation for any part you do not have adequate communication. Ideally, you should use an objective translator such as the AT&T translation service. However, I realize that this may not be financially viable for individual physicians in an office setting. In fact, the AT&T bill likely costs more than the patient charge.

However, physicians working in a hospital setting who do not have official translators available have no excuse not to use the AT&T service. Actually, because of JCAHO recommendations, every hospital must have translation available at the hospital's expense.

Besides official translators (e.g., an internal medicine physician who does not understand Spanish working in a high Spanish-speaking population area might decide it is worthwhile to hire a dedicated translator), there are other options. Some are better than others.

I can recall instances in medical school, before the JCAHO ruling, where the housekeeping staff often did double duty as translators for us. Clearly, this is not ideal. However, with no other options available, it was better than nothing.

There is certainly a temptation to use family members as translators. Again, in an office setting, this is likely the usual mode of obtaining information from non–English-speaking patients. There are some pitfalls of doing this: (1) Just because family members can speak English does not mean they can adequately translate medical terminology; (2) Family members may deliberately not translate accurately so as to downplay the disease process to their family member.

Also, some patients leave translation up to their children. Although their 9-year-old child may be very mature, for obvious reasons, he or she is not the best candidate with which to use to understand your patient.

In my lawsuit, I was fortunate that I gave the very critical discharge instructions using a hospital translator. Still, I anticipated the issue of communication with a non–English-speaking patient as becoming a potential source of damage for my case. Knowing your strengths and potential weaknesses is critical for a successful lawsuit.

In conclusion, language difficulties are one of the major communication issues with your patient, which represent potential sources for liability. Doing what you can to minimize these issues will help prevent a lawsuit.

> Patients who do not speak English still deserve a chance to communicate. Failure to do so can lead to misdiagnosis and a malpractice lawsuit.

Communication of informed consent

Informed consent is a discussion between doctor and patient whereby the doctor must explain to the patient, preparatory to a procedure, of the most common risks, complications, alternatives, and benefits. In some states, the test of whether proper informed consent was given is "would a reasonable person in the place of the plaintiff have agreed to the procedure, had they been advised of the same things in the same way." In some other states it is different, "whether this particular patient would have given consent."

Many physicians explain the procedure, use a fill-in form, and have the patient sign it. Although documentation of the informed consent is critical (and is discussed in more detail in Chapter 13), proper communication of the risks is imperative. Patients want to believe you and are optimistic that they will have a successful result. You have the power, in how you present the risks and benefits, to sway the patient toward or away from a particular procedure. However, patients must be consciously aware of the possibility of failure.

> In informed consent as in all documentation, the more you write the better. Do more than simply fill in the form.

As patients often forget these conversations of informed consent, it is wise to have family members present who will act as witness to your discussions. It is also advisable to have healthcare professionals act as witness to the signed informed consent. This gives you an added measure of protection. Clearly, good documentation is imperative to a strong defense. Chapter 13 has more information on documentation issues.

Chapter 13 **Good documentation makes a difference**

I have seen a lot said and written about the fact that good documentation will prevent a lawsuit. I disagree. Good documentation can go a long way to getting a defendant's verdict at trial. It might even be able to help you get your case dismissed. But good documentation rarely prevents someone from being sued.

Poor documentation can sink a case.

Nevertheless, good documentation *is* the cornerstone of a strong defense. But what is considered good documentation? There is a myth perpetuated amongst many physicians that the "less is more" tactic applies to their documentation. By this logic, the less you write, the less that can be twisted around and used against you.

However, juries perceive this differently. In an example of a missed brain bleed like a subarachnoid hemorrhage, it is better to mention something about it in your documentation. From the jury's point of view, it is better to consider something, use your judgment, and be wrong, than not to consider something at all. Judgment calls usually lean toward the defense.

However, careless doctors who do not even consider a brain bleed end up with plaintiff's verdicts. Therefore, abandon the "less is more" guidance for chart documentation. Instead, realize that the more you write, the better it is for your case.

Regarding documentation, it should go without saying, but I will say it anyway because of its extreme importance: *never alter your chart*. Anytime you retroactively buff your chart, it will come back to haunt you.

How to Survive a Medical Malpractice Lawsuit. By © Ilene R. Brenner. Published 2010 Blackwell Publishing, ISBN: 978-1-4443-3130-1.

Whatever you think might be damaging, and you feel the need to change, is actually very defensible compared to an altered chart. Good attorneys can make bad charts appear good. Nobody can repair the damage to a case once it is revealed that you altered the chart.

Sometimes, there are mistakes that were made in documentation that you noticed long before any claim was made against you. You are permitted to correct mistakes by two methods: (1) draw one line through it, write the word "error," then time and date the alteration and/or (2) add a separate addendum. Once a claim is made, however, no addendums should be added.

> Never, never, never alter your chart.

There is another circumstance that deserves mention. For instance, it is possible, even likely, that your carefully prepared chart can be lost by the billers and/or medical records department. Most facilities will inform you of charts that have not yet been completed. And it is usually part of your responsibilities to your employer and/or the hospital to have fully completed charting.

If you have a situation where you are being told to prepare a chart for a patient you no longer remember, months after rendering your care, do so only if you feel you can honestly recreate a chart based on available materials at your disposal.

In this special situation, you would be better-off having minimal documentation that would lead to under-billing the patient than to have a chart that could be misconstrued as falsified. In fact, for legal purposes, it might be better to avoid any delayed charting whatsoever and leave the documentation incomplete. This is especially true if that patient had a bad outcome and could possibly lead to a lawsuit.

Documentation of informed consent

Many cases are won or lost on the issue of informed consent. Some can even be prevented and/or dropped if excellent documentation of informed consent is given. As was mentioned earlier, when a patient needs a procedure performed, there are forms to fill out that are evidence that the patient gave informed consent for the doctor to perform the particular procedure.

Some doctors relegate this important part of their patient's care to a nurse or physician extender. Although I understand you may feel pressed for time, do not allow someone else to give the informed consent. Informed consent is a lot more than signing a form. This is a critical part of proper communication with your patient. You should explain to the patient the procedure and its most likely side effects, while still having them sign a form. Do not just do this in medical jargon. Use layman's terms, diagrams, and whatever else is necessary to fully explain what is about to happen.

If you and/or the hospital have standardized forms, make liberal use of underlines, circles, and insertions on the form (handwritten pictures and/or diagrams as mentioned earlier can be done here as well). Any personalization you add to a preprinted form will show that you made a deliberate effort to explain those risks to the patient.

Also, just because the hospital has a patient sign a form does not mean you do not have your own as well. As you are likely aware, patients often do not pay attention to you the first time you explain to them the risks and benefits. They tend to be in denial of any bad outcome possibilities, as they only want a good result.

Therefore, the more supporting documentation you have about informed consent, the better. This includes witnesses. These witnesses can be family members, nurses, and other staff members. If nurses have their own charting, make sure they were present during informed consent and have them create documentation to that effect.

In your chart, make sure you summarize your informed consent as well. However, give more details than a simple, "informed consent was given." The more explicit you are in your charting, the more believable you are to a jury.

It may seem repetitive, but the more times you perform informed consent, the better. And the more times it is referred to inside the chart, the better still. Juries will think you are a very careful doctor when they see so many instances where you documented your informed consent.

Some doctors go so far as to tape-record (with their patients' full knowledge and consent) the whole informed consent episode. Then, when a patient sues you for a bad outcome you never told them about, you will have undeniable proof. Different people go to different lengths to protect themselves.

If you have a diary, destroy it now before you get sued!

I know of a number of physicians who keep a diary. It can be personal or medical diaries. For some, it is a log of their life experience. For others, it is a list of the patients and their medical problems for informational, book research, or follow-up purposes.

Why are diaries bad? Anything that has dates can be used as evidence against you. Let us just say you log in your diary going out for drinks with friends. Then, years later you are sued, and the plaintiff's attorney discovers your "drinking orgy" the night before you treated their client. I can assure you they will use this information to paint you as a physician just steps from requiring the Talbott Recovery Campus.

If you are a physician who likes to keep detailed logs of your patients, have you followed HIPAA protocol? If not, I am sure the plaintiff's attorney will use that fact against you. Also, you cannot anticipate how your innocent log can be twisted out of context to hurt you.

Therefore, if you have any kind of diary, throw it away now. Also, cease keeping private logs of your patients beyond a few months. Ideally, you should not keep any private logs of your patients. The less the plaintiff's attorney can find to impeach you, the better.

If you insist on keeping a log of your interesting patients for future use in a book, then eliminate the use of names and dates and stick to generalities.

Also, realize there are other kinds of "diaries" such as your online diaries. Do you have a blog, facebook account, or twitter account? Depending on your jurisdiction, the plaintiff's attorney could ask you for all your passwords and search through these sites to find evidence for something that you have said that they could use against you. I will not say you cannot use these modern forms of communication. Just realize that anything you write or post, especially on patients and medical topics, could end up being read aloud in court. Therefore, be professional when online, and before you blog or twitter something, think to yourself, "How will this sound read aloud to a jury?"

Anything that you say publicly, whether through a comment feed or tweet, is searchable and can potentially be used against you in court. Also, realize that sites such as Sermo and Ozmosis are not peer-review protected, and those "innocent" opinions that you give on case studies could be used by the plaintiff attorney if your lawsuit happens to be on one of those topics. For instance, you say one thing in your deposition but have a different opinion on Sermo. That could put you in a difficult situation where the plaintiff's attorney accuses you of lying in your deposition.

Another point, be careful when using the Internet at work. Many hospitals track and archive your use, and a savvy plaintiff's attorney could subpoena these records and identify personal and medical websites you accessed before (or even during) your patient's care. Be cognizant that you have an electronic footprint that could possibly be traced and then used against you. Some states are more liberal than others in regard to what can be used in court.

> Be careful about your electronic footprint on the web, in particular, any non–peer-review protected opinions you give on medical cases.

My advice may seem weird now, perhaps even extreme, but in 2 or 3 years from now, when a doctor is sued, these issues will likely be more commonplace as plaintiff's attorneys get more familiar with social media. Physicians need to be warned of the future or else the mistakes they make now could perhaps be used against them when that lawsuit comes to pass.

Rulebook: Social media for physicians:
- Use social media as a communication tool, not a diagnostic tool.
- Be careful about commenting on case presentations on sites such as Sermo and Ozmosis. Your opinion can (in many jurisdictions) be used against you in court.
- Imagine everything you write as being read aloud to a jury.
- Do not assume anonymity. In some locations, you can be requested to give your IDs and passwords for public social media accounts.

Be legible

Physicians are famous for their poor handwriting. Although you do not have to excel in penmanship, having illegible documentation can hurt you at trial. How can you defend yourself if nobody can read what you wrote? Often, physicians who can read and interpret their handwriting soon after creating an entry cannot read it months or years later.

Therefore, if you know that there is no hope in improving your handwriting, it is best you use alternate forms of documentation. Dictation is very popular among doctors. Computerized documentation is also increasing in popularity. Many physicians use scribes for both legibility and productivity. In this era of high technology, there is no excuse to have illegible records.

Read what you document

A big part of good documentation is using these valuable notations. When you see a patient for a follow-up visit from a recent hospital stay, it is imperative that you review the hospital records. If you have a new patient, you must request and examine the previous treating physician's records. And when patients come to you for their 10th visit, you should be aware of what occurred on the previous 9 examinations. What good is all this valuable documentation if you do not read it?

From a legal perspective, a jury expects that physicians will access any information that is available to them to assist in the patient's diagnosis.

The jury will not accept an explanation of having a busy practice or incompetent staff. Emergency physicians, because of the nature of their job, are typically given more leeway with this. All other physicians are expected to have made an informed decision when establishing a diagnosis and treatment plan. If you fail to do this, and the patient is misdiagnosed, your defensible error in judgment becomes medical malpractice.

Reading documentation is as important as writing it.

Physicians can make errors in judgment that are later construed as malpractice, however, there is much within the physician's control to optimize the risk factors that can lead to a lawsuit, such as good communication and documentation. However, when physicians hire mid-level providers (MLPs) such as nurse practitioners and physicians assistants, a degree of control over the process is lost. Chapter 14 examines these complex issues of liability with regard to the use of MLPs.

Chapter 14 **Liability risk with the use of physician extenders**

Can you be sued for the malpractice of one of your physician extenders?

The short answer is yes. However, it is not as clear-cut as you might think. Of course, you can be sued for anything. But what is the liability risk?

Whether or not you agree with the movement toward practice of medicine without direct physician supervision, physician extenders such as physician assistants (PAs) and nurse practitioners (NPs) have become a modern reality. Retail stores such as CVS and Wal-Mart are establishing in-store "walk in" clinics that employ mid-level providers (MLPs) who practice without direct physician oversight. In fact, emergency departments across the country have fast tracks run by MLPs.

Although laws vary by state, several common elements govern the care that an MLP may legally provide. MLPs may perform a history and physical examination, and most states allow MLPs to diagnose medical conditions. About half of the states give "NPs" the explicit authority to order tests. Many states allow MLPs to prescribe medicines, including restricted drugs, without requiring a cosignature from a physician, although only a few states grant MLPs prescriptive authority without physician involvement.

Some states such as Alaska, New Hampshire, and Washington allow NPs to practice independently without any oversight by a physician. However, most states require that MLPs establish a "collaborative agreement" with a physician that spells out the MLP's scope of practice. The contents of a collaborative agreement are subject to state laws and may vary based on the MLP's experience and knowledge, as well as any limits of hospital by-laws (if a hospital-based MLP).

How to Survive a Medical Malpractice Lawsuit. By © Ilene R. Brenner. Published 2010 Blackwell Publishing, ISBN: 978-1-4443-3130-1.

> Physician extenders can not only be individually liable for their actions but also increase your own liability.

MLPs may be individually liable if they exceed their scope of practice. For example, MLPs who attempt to manage a hypotensive patient with an acute abdomen but who do not seek guidance from their supervising physician may be held liable for exceeding their scope of practice.

Physicians may be held liable for the actions of MLPs under several circumstances.

Inadequate supervision

In the states that allow independent MLP practice, the collaborative agreement that defines the extender's scope of practice and specific supervisory duties is the key to determine the physician liability. In this case, your duties could be as simple as being available for consult and signing and reviewing the extender's charts.

In the states that do not allow MLPs to practice independently, the state Medical Practice Acts will require that the supervising physician maintains the final responsibility for the care of the patient and the performance of the PA. In this case, *the physician could bear significant liability for any errors committed by the MLP.*

Improper delegation of authority

Some states require a written description of the authority delegated to MLPs. If a physician is found to have delegated too much authority to an MLP based on that MLP's education and training, the physician may also be subject to liability. For example, in *Gillis v. Cardio TVP Surgical Associates* (520 S.E. 2d 767), the Georgia Court of Appeals stated that physicians do not have "carte blanche to delegate any and all tasks to an assistant" and that a jury would have to decide whether a PA had "the requisite skill level and training" to perform a vein harvest surgery that ultimately resulted in an injury to a patient.

Vicarious liability

Vicarious liability is a legal concept that essentially says that you can be liable for the actions of your employees and partners. If a physician employs an MLP, then the physician could be vicariously liable for the actions of the MLP. Similarly, if the physician is a partner in a group that employs MLPs, depending on the structure of the group, the physician partner could be subject to liability for the negligence of the group's employee. However, if you are a physician employee of a medical group, you are not vicariously liable for the actions of an MLP.

It is more difficult to impose liability upon physicians for the actions of independent contractor MLPs, although liability may still be imposed under the theory of "apparent agency" when independent contractors act in a manner that makes a patient believe that the independent contractor is the physician's agent. For example, if an independent contractor MLP wears a coat containing the physician practice's logo and introduces himself as "Dr. Welby's physician assistant," liability could still be imposed despite the PA's independent contractor status.

An example

It is very common to have physician extenders work independently in the fast-track of an emergency department. Many practices have the emergency physicians review and sign the charts of the MLPs who were working during their shift, although they never saw the MLPs at any time during their shift and may not have received any calls from them either. This understandably makes the physicians required to sign these charts uncomfortable about the liability risk.

> In many states, physician extenders do not need direct physician supervision and can write prescriptions without cosignature.

Let me clarify the word *liability*. There is a legal definition as mentioned in the *Glossary*. There is also a more commonly used term *liability risk* that people often use interchangeable but more accurately refers to ability to be sued. The best practice to reduce the likelihood of being sued is to always see the patient yourself. Your state may permit the aforementioned scenario, and a judge in summary judgment or jury at trial may agree that you followed the law—both federal and state. However, following the law will not prevent you from getting sued because your name is on the chart. As I have already stated that the moment physicians are sued, they have already lost on some level; your goal is to try to prevent a lawsuit.

Some physicians are uncomfortable with the fact that they are signing a chart because billing rules require a physician's signature on every chart despite the fact that the physician extenders practiced independently. Payers typically require the signature as proof that supervisory conditions were met even though supervision can simply mean that you were available in the department or through phone consult. Many physicians seek to make it clear to a plaintiff's attorney reviewing your chart that they did not see the patient and only signed the chart for billing reasons in an attempt to prevent getting sued or minimize that risk. They sometimes write in some kind of qualifier to that effect.

In my opinion, any time your name is on a chart you can be pulled into a lawsuit. However, the following statement has been suggested to me for physicians who insist on writing something on their chart: "this chart is being signed for billing purposes only, and is in accordance with state and federal laws."

How should you run your practice?

First, learn the laws in your state that apply to MLPs. Once you are familiar with the laws, you can decide how much authority to delegate to the MLPs.

> Every state has different laws about physician extenders and their scope of practice.

If you are placed in a supervisory role, it must be clearly delineated what the collaborating physician's responsibilities will be. Regardless of what state you practice in, you must be comfortable with the extent (or limitations) of each MLP's scope of practice.

In addition, just as with other employees, MLPs should have regular performance evaluations and employee education. As physician extenders can be individually liable, it is critical that any MLP you supervise carries adequate malpractice insurance.

Whether you allow the MLP to work independently under your supervision depends on your comfort level. A larger company may feel more comfortable shouldering the risk of this practice. A smaller company may not. If you are a company (or partner), you must weigh the monetary benefits of the increased productivity created by the MLPs versus the costs of litigation incurred by lawsuits for vicarious liability.

In fact, a smaller physician group who is looking for extra coverage and trying to decide between an extra physician versus MLPs might decide that the complex risks of physician extenders outweighs the increased cost of the extra physician.

And when deciding whether to work for a company that employs independently practicing MLPs, you too have to consider the risks. You have to decide for yourself whether the benefit of independent physician extenders outweighs the potential for being drawn into a lawsuit that may eventually get dismissed.

There are no easy answers to this question. Unfortunately, the use of MLPs introduces extra variables that can make preventing a lawsuit for a bad outcome difficult to impossible. This is not very reassuring when the goal is not only to win your case but also to not get sued in the first place.

Being aware of the potentials for liability will help make a team approach to medical practice rewarding for all involved. Hospitals, too, have complex interactions with physicians that affect physician liability. Chapter 15 has more information on this important topic.

Chapter 15 **Hospital issues**

Peer review

In this age of increased attention to quality and accountability in medicine, there has been a quandary created by competing interests: How can healthcare organizations and their physicians share valuable data about errors and judgment issues to improve care without opening themselves up to a lawsuit?

Thus, the legal concept of peer review was born. A peer review committee may be responsible for: (1) evaluating and improving the quality of care given; (2) reviewing credentials of healthcare providers applying or reapplying for hospital privileges; and (3) investigating allegations against healthcare provider.

The legal statutes state that the proceedings, findings, and records of peer review committees are protected from discovery and are normally inadmissible as evidence in judicial or administrative proceedings, and all 50 states plus the District of Columbia have enacted peer review statutes that provide varying degrees of immunity (Beall, 1998).

Online sites such as Sermo and Ozmosis review cases but are not subject to protection by peer review. Be careful while giving medical opinions there.

There may be times you work on a hospital committee and specific patient cases are discussed. It is imperative that if you discuss specific cases, you do so within the confines of peer review. If not, the notes from that meeting can be subpoenaed for use at trial.

How to Survive a Medical Malpractice Lawsuit. By © Ilene R. Brenner. Published 2010 Blackwell Publishing, ISBN: 978-1-4443-3130-1.

> If your administrator or colleague wishes to discuss a patient, make sure it is in a true peer review setting.

Hospital privileges

When you fill out paperwork to be credentialed at a hospital, you receive a form that asks what are the procedures in which you are capable. How you handle this form can contribute to winning or losing a case in which a procedure you perform becomes an issue.

> Don't do anything not explicitly stated in your hospital privileges. Period.

The procedures you list should be things you are confident about performing and approved by your appropriate specialty board. For instance, you may be an internist who took a weekend course teaching Botox™ and skin biopsies. However, if the internal medicine board does not have a policy supporting the use of these procedures by their members, you could be at risk if sued for malpractice in the event these procedures led to a bad outcome. You may feel completely able in performing these procedures, check them off, and even get them approved by a hospital. However, in court, the plaintiff's attorney will have a dermatologist or plastic surgeon who will detail all the months and years of training he or she had to be properly skilled in these procedures, and without your own board having a specific policy supporting you, the jury will most likely see that your training was substandard and that the bad outcome is a result of your inadequate training.

> Do not try to get credentialed for procedures not sanctioned by your board.

I know of a case where a pediatric cardiovascular surgeon performed bypass surgery on an adult, who suffered a severe complication and died. The jury felt that while the surgeon had been trained to do bypass surgeries on adults and children, they performed so few on adults that their skills were inadequate and ruled for the plaintiff with a multimillion-dollar verdict. The hospital had granted privileges to this physician, but multiple experts verified what a typical layperson would assume, which is that pediatric specialists should not work with adults.

Conversely, just because your board approves of a procedure, it does not mean you should check it off. For instance, you may work at a hospital where radiologists place PICC lines for IV access, and surgeons place central lines for after-hours emergency venous access. If you are an emergency physician practicing in this environment for many years, and have not had some kind of course to keep your central line placement skills active, you should not check that off on the privileges sheet as a competence. Or if you feel comfortable doing femoral lines but not subclavian lines, you should specify that distinction.

Risk management: Does it help you?

If you in some capacity work in a hospital environment, you should have had some interaction with risk management. The most common circumstance is peer review. Risk management usually runs the quality assurance of the medical departments to ensure that whatever is discussed is legally protected under peer review statutes.

However, there are many other reasons why you might hear from risk management. One peculiar situation I experienced was with a patient I had under close observation by security for a psychotic break. When the portable X-ray machine rolled into his room, he declared the intentions of the government to infect his mind through that apparatus and freaked out. Security lapsed and the patient fled into the local neighborhood. The police found him jumping on top of a car, and they brought him back into our care (with some new injuries). Risk management wanted to know my opinion as to whether I thought the hospital was at fault for his injuries and whether they should pay for the damage to the car. However, I realized what they were really asking me was if subpoenaed by an attorney, how would I testify?

In another instance, risk management showed me a letter they received from an attorney for a patient I saw. It was a demand for money from the hospital. It detailed a list of the hospital's and my "deficiencies." Risk management wanted me to defend myself and wanted to know whether the hospital deficiencies had merit.

I realize now that I should not have said anything and should have deferred to my attorney. However, I gave my opinion that the plaintiff's attorney's allegations did not even make medical sense. I also said that the hospital did have a role in the patient's poor outcome, and they should consider settling before the inevitable lawsuit was initiated by the plaintiff.

Again, risk management was fishing for the hospital. They wanted to know whether the complaint had merit, and how would I be as a potential witness against the hospital?

What is the lesson in this? Risk management is there to protect the hospital. You should be very wary when dealing with risk management. Outside of peer review, you should not discuss anything with risk management unless your attorney is involved.

If risk management confronts you about a patient, find out as much information as you can: for example, name of patient, date seen, and issues being brought up. However, if asked about your opinions, first tell risk management you need to see a copy of the chart (and make a note of the specifics in case you never get a hard copy), then inform them you cannot make any statements regarding this patient outside the presence of your own private attorney. Next, call the insurance company to report this patient as a potential claim and ask to have representation assigned to you (or if you already have a relationship with an approved defense attorney, ask to get them assigned to you) to run interference for you with risk management.

The against medical advice form

I am sure you think that patient's signing this form absolves you of all liability if something goes wrong. It does not. Worse, horrible things happen to patients who sign out against medical advice (AMA). When they die, their surviving relatives will not look kindly upon the physician who allowed their relative to leave the hospital when it was clear that they were sick. Although you cannot stop some patients from leaving the emergency department, you should do your best to convince them to stay.

Some people express their anxiety about being sick by acting out in anger. They have a short fuse and get frustrated easily. And frustrated patients often lead to aggravated physicians who wish the patients would just "go away." At these times, physicians often are relieved when a nurse comes by saying, "The patient wants to sign out AMA." Do not just let it happen. Take a deep breath, walk in their room, and ask the patient in a calm voice if there is anything that you can do to get them to stay. Do they need pain medicine? Do they want to smoke? Or need something that can help relax them? If letting them go smoke or putting a nicotine patch on their arm will help get them to stay, do it. For the patient's sake and for your own decreased liability.

Also, what are the issues behind the patient wanting to leave? Sometimes, the patient feels sick, comes to the hospital, waits five hours to be seen, and now the babysitter has to leave and there is no one to take care of the kids. Or they have to show up in court. There can be many reasons why they need to leave. I have had many situations where the patient came in thinking you were going to give them a prescription, but you feel they were sick enough to get admitted, but the patient just cannot drop their life and come into the hospital. Some people need a day to get their affairs in order to get admitted.

The key is to show patients compassion. Even angry patients will have a hard time criticizing the doctor who cares too much about the patient's welfare to willingly discharge them AMA. If patients refuse to stay, see if they will agree to come back later. I have had a number of patients who left the hospital and 8 h later when they ran their errands (such as receiving and cashing their monthly check) came back for their abscess drainage or cardiac monitoring for angina. Call their personal doctor to convince them to stay. If the patients give you permissions to release you from a HIPAA violation, call their mother, girlfriend, wife, children, close friend, or pastor to discuss the situation with the patients and talk sense into them. Always leave the door open for their return. Make them feel welcome enough to want to come back again.

It is inevitable that you will have ignorant patients who make poor decisions but unfortunately are mentally competent enough to leave the hospital if they wish. However, you must have witnesses and fantastic documentation. You must be able to prove that you tried everything in your power to talk them out of leaving.

I have seen a number of physicians sign the AMA form as a witness. Don't. You are the physician treating the patient. The witness should be a close family member ideally. Otherwise, friends or hospital staff should be used as the witness. It is a conflict of interest for you to be the treating physician and the witness of the signing of the AMA form. Also, do not allow the form to be your only documentation. In some states, the only legal AMA documentation is a note in the chart. Whether you fill out a form or not, make sure to make notations in the chart that confirm the patient had the mental capacity to make a decision, why they need to stay, who you told (patient, family, friends, etc.), who witnessed it, and a summary of your efforts to talk the patient into staying. Also, ask the nurse to document your discussions with the patient as well.

Also, a former colleague of mine tells me that his hospital calls all patients who left AMA in a day or two to check on their progress and once again impress upon the patient the importance of returning to the hospital. This is an excellent technique to both help patient satisfaction and decrease your liability. And you can help with your patients' health too, as studies show that more than 20% of patients who leave AMA actually required admission to the hospital.

If patients are impaired, mentally incompetent, and unable to make a proper decision for their care (e.g., in Georgia, if a patient is declared that they are a danger to themselves or others, this could vary by state), you cannot allow them to leave the hospital AMA. Under these circumstances, it is imperative that you declare them incompetent for their own good.

You might have to use chemical and physical restraints to do this. You certainly will need to document the heck out of the encounter to prove that these patients are mentally incompetent and unable to make their own decisions. Impaired patients who are allowed to sign out AMA and then have a bad outcome will likely lead to lawsuits.

Do not allow yourself to have your privileges suspended

How many doctors have charts that are delinquent? A lot. How many hospitals have a number of physicians at any given time on suspension for failure to do proper documentation on a patient? A lot. As this is so common, you might think it is not a big deal. However, it is.

The plaintiff's attorney will ask if you have ever had your hospital privileges suspended or revoked. Even though you will have some opportunity to explain that the suspension was "just for a medical records issue," juries may not see this as insignificant. After all, your care is being judged in this court of law. Careless doctors, who allow incomplete medical records to cause them to get suspended, might just be careless enough to have caused medical malpractice to this patient. Juries take this issue very seriously. So should you.

So much of what physicians do every day is fraught with danger—to their patients and to their career. Certainly, it is important to assess the risks and benefits when determining the appropriate treatment for your patients. It is no less essential for the physician to be aware of the potential pitfalls of what appear to be mundane procedures such as informed consent and medical record-keeping.

Furthermore, it is widely quoted that the best defense is a good offense. I wrote this book with the intention of helping physicians prevent, prepare, and succeed in their medical malpractice lawsuit. The next and final chapter is a summary with the most important points of the book listed in a quick-fire fashion, which, along with the book in its entirety, will give you the power you need to be your own best advocate.

Reference

Beall D. Protecting resident performance evaluations under peer review immunity law. JAMA 1998;280(2):192.

Chapter 16 **Summary**

As you can see, the process of a medical malpractice lawsuit is a long road fraught with danger at every turn. However, it is my hope that by reading this book, you are now prepared to handle what is otherwise a confusing and frustrating experience. In this chapter, a summary of the process, highlighting the most critical aspects of a lawsuit, is provided.

1 You receive a subpoena.
   a) Call your insurance company and make sure you know the basics of your insurance policy such as limits, consent to settle clause, and ability to choose your own attorney.
   b) Do not look up any information in a book, journal, or online until you have met with your attorney.
   c) Do not destroy or alter evidence.
2 Four criteria make up a successful claim against a physician.
   a) duty
   b) breach
   c) proximate cause
   d) damages
   Although getting your case settled through alternative dispute resolution can save the stress of a lawsuit, realize that any payments made will be reported to the National Practitioner Data Bank.
3 Evaluate your attorney using the questions listed in Chapter 3.
   a) Is there a conflict of interest? Not satisfied with your attorney? If so you need to switch attorneys.
   b) If you think you need your own attorney separate from your codefendants:
      – Ask the insurance company representative.
      – If they refuse, keep making noise with their superiors.
      – Use the term "conflict of interest" liberally.
      – Ask your attorney to recuse themselves if you still are not successful.

How to Survive a Medical Malpractice Lawsuit. By © Ilene R. Brenner. Published 2010 Blackwell Publishing, ISBN: 978-1-4443-3130-1.

  – Last resort, threaten to sue your attorney for legal malpractice.
  – Put all your requests in writing.
4 Are you tired, angry, frustrated, anxious, or depressed (or a combination thereof)? Remember to try the following to keep your head in the game to help yourself to be the best defendant possible.
  a) pay attention to your attorney
  b) focus on your case
  c) be objective
  d) learn to play the game
  e) Ask for help
5 Nail the deposition.
  a) Get as much training as possible. Ask for a preparation specialist. This is one of the most critical aspects of your case.
  b) Know your strategy for dealing with codefendants.
  c) Make sure you understand well the basic medicine components to your case.
  d) Dress appropriately.
  e) Treat the questions in a business-like manner.
  f) Be confident.
  g) Do not interrupt the questioner.
  h) Use "medicalese" generously.
  i) Answering questions. Beware of certain traps: rule out, double negatives, compound questions, statements that precede the actual question, and hypotheticals.
  j) The less you say, the better.
6 Can your case be dismissed? Ask your attorney if your case is a good candidate for a motion for summary judgment.
7 Wait.
  a) There will be long periods of time where nothing happens with your case.
8 The trial date approaches: Prepare.
  a) Know your deposition inside and out.
  b) Become an expert on the medicine. Know every statistic and where they come from. Know all the current research.
  c) Identify your weaknesses and make them strengths.
  d) Get ready for your cross-examination. Try to get a trial preparation specialist who will help you. Do sample question and answer sessions in front of a video camera to see how you look to a jury.
9 The trial.
  a) Listen to your attorney.
  b) Be professional.

c) Dress appropriately.

d) Never talk about the case in public areas outside of the courtroom.

e) Practice your poker face and do not show emotion during the various events at trial.

f) On your cross-examination: Do not be too quick to agree with the plaintiff's attorney. Answer a question with a question. Be ready to summarize your whole case in a few quick sentences. Be wary of any questions that ask whether you agree with something. Stay cool at all times. Do not parry with the attorney. Look at the jury when answering questions. Never sound condescending. Use the three-second rule when answering questions. Beware of anything given to you by plaintiff's attorney to look at on the stand, use layman's terms at all times when answering questions. Make sure you know your deposition verbatim.

g) Do not lie.

h) Do not fidget in court.

i) If you win, be professional and accept your victory with dignity.

10 If you lose.

a) Find out if there are grounds for an appeal, and if your insurance company has agreed to pursue one.

11 Do whatever you can to prevent a lawsuit—try to minimize the likelihood of the two essential elements creating a lawsuit: a bad outcome or an angry patient (or their family).

a) Bad outcome: Most patients fall within statistical norms for adverse events. However, if you are outside of the norm, or are finding your care repeatedly deemed negligent in peer review, you need to look within and ask yourself if you can improve your patient care.

b) Angry patients: Much of the issues are communication related.

– Show compassion, act like you care, listen to your patients, and treat them with respect.

– Be available to your patients, spend time with them, and do not always pass them off on your physician extender.

– Do not waste your patients' time. If you know you are running late, have your office make an attempt to notify your patients through phone/email/text message.

12 Avoid common pitfalls in communication that can lead to a lawsuit or harm your chances of winning.

a) It is not what you say, but what patients hear. Repetition is key. Ask your patients to repeat back your instructions to ensure their correct understanding.

b) Get a proper translator for patients who speak a foreign language.

   c) Document the patient's informed consent in detail, with personalization, multiple witnesses, and redundant notations by the nurse and you in multiple locations.

   d) If something goes wrong, an apology can go a long way to preventing a lawsuit. (Be aware of the "I'm Sorry" laws in your state to know if this could be held against you in court as an admission against interest.)

13 Poor documentation can sink your case.

   a) The more you write, the better. Show your thought process in arriving at your diagnosis. List all the consultants you talked to or attempted to reach, with the number of times called by you, returned by them, and the details of the conversation.

   b) Never alter your chart.

   c) Document informed consent thoroughly.

   d) If you have not yet been sued, and have a patient log or diary, destroy it! If you are thinking about creating one, do not. If you insist on writing a log for future use in a book, eliminate the use of names and dates and stick to generalities.

   e) Be careful about anything you write in a blog, on twitter, and on a sites such as Sermo and Ozmosis.

   f) Be legible.

   g) Read your own and other physician's documentation.

14 Other potential pitfalls.

   a) Be cognizant of the risks of using physician extenders in your practice as you could be vicariously liable for their actions if you are an employer/partner.

   b) Use the peer review statute to your advantage, but do not be fooled by hospital settings that seem like peer review, but are not, and thus, do not offer your legal protections for any discussions that take place.

   c) Pay close attention to the procedures you apply for when you get credentialed at your hospital. Do not try to get credentialed for procedures not sanctioned by your board or that you do not have familiarity with any longer.

   d) Be wary when risk management attempts to discuss patients outside of peer review and outside the presence of your own attorney. Risk management is there to protect the hospital. Not you.

   e) Be cautious when using the against medical advice form.

   f) Do not be careless with your medical record-keeping. If you allow yourself to get suspended for delinquent medical records, it can be used against you in court. And regardless of how meaningless you think it is, juries take this issue very seriously.

Appendix A **Expert qualification requirements vary by state**

In the below sections I parse out the states that have strict or loose qualification requirements for experts. Some states have no requirements for experts at all, assuming that any lay person on a jury can comprehend the issues regardless of special training. Others simply require an expert be a licensed physician. Some are stricter and require that the expert have training in the issue at hand. However, the strictest requirements specify that the expert must have the same training as the defendant physician.

States with stringent expert qualification laws

The following states have laws that require the plaintiff's expert to be in the same specialty. This is most often determined by licensure in the appropriate regulatory board, trained and experienced in the same specialty, certified by an appropriate American board in the same specialty, and has practiced in this specialty recently. Any special rules will be noted:

Alabama – Requires practice in the same specialty during the year preceding the date that the alleged breach of standard of care occurred.

Arizona – Requires active practice in the same specialty as a majority of their professional time or instruction of students in the same specialty for the year immediately preceding the occurrence giving rise to the lawsuit.

Arkansas

Colorado – An exception for same specialty is made if the expert is in a field that is similar to the defendant and that the standards of care and practice in the two fields are similar.

Georgia – Adopted the Daubert Standard in civil cases.

How to Survive a Medical Malpractice Lawsuit. By © Ilene R. Brenner. Published 2010 Blackwell Publishing, ISBN: 978-1-4443-3130-1.

Kansas – Expert must devote at least 50% of their professional time, within a two-year period preceding the incident, to actual clinical practice in the same profession as defendant.

Michigan – Expert must have any board certifications that the defendant has.

New Jersey – During the year immediately preceeding the date of the occurrence, the expert must have devoted a majority of their professional time to the active clinical practice, or teaching of medicine.

South Carolina – Expert must be licensed and maintain board certification in the same specialty as the defendant. Also, the expert must have actively practiced or taught in the area of specialty for three of the last five years immediately preceding the opinion.

States with weak expert qualification laws

The following states have weak laws regarding experts. Some don't have any specific statutes regarding expert qualifications.

Alaska, California, Delaware, D.C., Hawaii, Idaho, Iowa, Kentucky, Maine, Maryland, Massachusetts, Minnesota

Mississippi – Expert simply needs to be a licensed physician.

Missouri, Nebraska, New Mexico, New York, North Dakota, Oklahoma, Oregon, Rhode, Island, South Dakota

Tennessee – Experts must be licensed in Tennessee or a contiguous bordering state and practicing for at least one year prior to the date of the plaintiff's injury.

Utah, Vermont, Washingtonk, Wisconsin, Wyoming

States with moderately stringent qualification laws

The following states have fairly stringent expert requirements; however, they allow for "similar" health care provider, with training in the issues pertinent to the claim. This is not as stringent as requirements to be in the "same" field of medicine as the defendant.

Connecticut – Requires a "similar health care provider" based on training, experience and knowledge as a result of practicing or teaching in a related field of medicine within the last five years. If the defendant is board certified, the expert must also be board certified.

Florida – Expert must practice in "same or similar" specialty as the defendant, and if a specialist, the expert must have practiced in the "same or similar" specialty for the past three years in active clinical practice, teaching, or in a clinical research program.

Illinois – Expert must be in the "same or substantially similar" medical specialty and must have actively practiced, taught, or done research in a university setting, for the past five years.

Montana – Expert must be in the same specialty as the defendant unless the standards of care and practice are substantially similar. Also, they must have treated, taught, or done clinical research for the diagnosis or condition at issue within the past five years.

Nevada – Expert must practice in a substantially similar area as defendant at the time of alleged negligence.

New Hampshire – The requirement for the expert to be competent and qualified to have rendered care when the alleged injury occurred was held to be unconstitutional.

North Carolina – Experts must be practicing or teaching in the same/similar specialty as the defendant.

Ohio – Experts must practice in the same or substantially similar specialty as the defendant and spend 75% of their professional time in clinical practice or teaching.

Pennsylvania – Experts must be in the same or similar specialty and board certified, if applicable, as the defendant.

Texas – Expert must be actively practicing and be board certified or have other substantive training or experience in an area of medical practice relevant to the claim.

Virginia – Expert must have specialized knowledge of the standards of care of defendants specialty and have active clinical practice in defendant's specialty or a related field of medicine within one year of the date of the alleged act or omission.

West Virginia – Expert must be currently trained and licensed to practice in the same or similar specialty.

The following states have pre-trial screening panels that determine the standard of care:

Indiana – Claims must be presented to a medical review panel prior to commencement of the action in court unless all parties issue a written waiver. The panel consists of one lawyer and three health care providers (no specific requirements are listed). The panel presents the expert opinion, which is admissible at trial but not conclusive. A plaintiff's attorney need not supply their own expert.

Louisiana – Providers insured by the Patient Compensation Fund are subject to a nonbinding medical review panel comprised of one nonvoting lawyer and three physicians (no specific requirements are listed). The panel issues a written opinion and their determinations constitute expert testimony.

References

American Medical Association (AMA), *Select State Laws II, Liability Reform.pdf*, February 2008, http://www.ama-assn.org

McCullough, Campbell & Lane LLP, *Summary of Medical Malpractice Law*, http://www.mcandl.com/states.html

American Tort Reform Association State and Federal Reforms, http://www.atra.org/reforms/

Expertlaw, *Medical Malpractice Law – A State By State Overview*, http://www.expertlaw.com/library/malpractice_by_state/

Onecle Court Opinions, *Texas Civil Practice & Remedies Code – Section 74.401, Qualifications of Expert Witness In Suit Against Physician*, http://law.onecle.com/texas/civil/74.401.00.html

LAWriter Ohio Laws and Rules, http://codes.ohio.gov/orc/2743.43

Appendix B **Arbitration, mediation, and pretrial screening panels**

Alternative dispute resolution: There are many methods, many are voluntary, some are mandatory, the results can be binding or nonbinding. Note: States can appear in more than one section.

States with arbitration

Alabama – Both parties must agree in writing, agreements are binding, irrevocable.

Alaska – Arbitration is voluntary and permitted in contracts if it is not a condition of providing services.

California – Arbitration is not mandated but is permitted.

Connecticut – Arbitration is not mandated but is permitted.

D.C. – Arbitration is permitted but not required. While arbitration can be a final judgment, parties can still seek judicial review, and evidence admitted in arbitration is admissible but can't be identified in court as being from arbitration.

Florida – Voluntary and binding. Also, a judge may refer cases to nonbinding arbitration.

Georgia – Arbitration is permitted but not required. It is binding only if the decision to arbitrate was made after a claim of alleged negligence occurred. The decision has an effect of a final judgment, and can be appealed to the Superior Court.

Hawaii – Mandatory medical claims conciliation panel that determines negligence, but either party can reject the decision and take the claim to court.

Idaho – Arbitration is permitted but not required. It is nonbinding and decisions are not admissible in court.

Illinois – Arbitration is not mandatory but is permitted. For amounts less than $50,000, the court may order aribitration.

How to Survive a Medical Malpractice Lawsuit. By © Ilene R. Brenner. Published 2010 Blackwell Publishing, ISBN: 978-1-4443-3130-1.

Kentucky – Arbitration agreements are voluntary and binding.

Louisiana – Arbitration is allowed but not mandated, and are binding. Any claims that are not taken to arbitration must be evaluated by a medical review panel.

Maryland – Arbitration is required but can be waived by any party to the action. Each side reserves the right to reject the arbitration decision and proceed to trial; however, the decision is admissible and presumed correct in court.

Michigan – Voluntary binding arbitration for damages less than $75,000.

Minnesota – Voluntary and nonbinding.

Mississippi – Voluntary and binding.

New Jersey – Mandatory for all cases in amounts of less than $20,000. The decision is nonbinding and inadmissible.

New York – Defendants may concede liability and agree to arbitration on damages. HMOs are authorized to have participants agree prior to treatment that all claims will be arbitrated.

North Carolina – Voluntary arbitration is capped at $1 million total damages.

North Dakota – Not binding, but some form of ADR must be attempted prior to filing a lawsuit.

Ohio – Permitted but not required, and nonbinding and inadmissible in court.

Pennsylvania – Mandatory arbitration is unconstitutional.

South Carolina – Parties may agree to binding arbitration.

South Dakota – Not mandated, but permitted. The arbitration panel makes a determination and then gives the parties 30 days to agree on damages. If the parties fail to agree, the panel will make a determination on damages.

Tennessee – Not mandated, but permitted.

Texas – Not mandated.

Utah – The mandatory pre-screening panel can be converted into binding arbitration.

Vermont – Mandatory, and the decision can be appealed unless parties agree that arbitration should be binding.

Virginia – Parties can agree to binding arbitration in advance of treatment; however, the plaintiff can opt out within 60 days after termination of treatment.

Washington – Voluntary binding arbitration is available.

States with mediation

Florida – Within 120 days after a suit is filed, all parties must attend mediation in person if binding arbitration has not already been agreed to.

Michigan – Mandatory mediation panel review. Each party may reject the decision, and if rejected, the case will proceed to trial. The rejecting party shall pay the other party's actual costs unless the verdict favors the rejecting party and/or the mediators decision was not unanimous.

North Carolina – Mediation can be ordered by the court, but findings are not admissible.

South Carolina – Before trial, some form of ADR must take place, which includes mediation that is governed by ADR rules.

Texas – Pre-trial mediation is routine in many venues. Nonbinding. Also, allowances have been made for mini-trials, moderated settlement conferences, and summary jury trials.

Washington – Mandatory but nonbinding.

West Virginia – Voluntary, confidential, and the decision is not admissible in court.

Wisconsin – Mandatory for claimants prior to commencing a suit, and the proceedings are not recorded and are inadmissible.

States with pretrial screening panels

Alaska – If arbitration does not occur, the court must appoint an advisory panel. The determination is admissible as evidence at trial.

Delaware – Any opinion by the panel is admissible as prima facie evidence at trial.

Florida – The pre-suit investigation process determines if there was negligence, and if so, the parties can elect to pursue arbitration for damages.

Hawaii – A medical claim reconciliation panel files an advisory opinion prior to commencement of a medical tort action in court. The decision is nonbinding and not admissible in court.

Idaho – The hearing panel decision is nonbinding and inadmissible at trial.

Indiana – At the request of either party, a medical review panel evaluates the case. At least two members must be of the same specialty as the defendant. The opinion is admissible at trial but not conclusive.

Kansas – The panel must be requested by one of the parties or upon a judge's own motion. The findings are admissible at trial.

Louisiana – Providers insured by the Patient Compensation Fund will have a mandatory medical review panel consisting of three physicians and one attorney. The report shall be admissible as evidence, but is not conclusive.

Maine – Mandatory pre-litigation screening panel, which consists of a physician, health care provider, and a chairperson. The findings are confidential.

Massachusetts – Every action for medical malpractice must be heard by a medical tribunal and the decision is admissible at trial.

Montana – Mandatory panel evaluation must occur prior to the filing of a claim. The decision is nonbinding and not admissible in court.

Nebraska – Mandatory evaluation by a medical review panel. The majority decision is submitted to the court; however, the majority and minority opinions may be submitted as evidence, and any panel member can be called as a witness.

Nevada – All parties must submit to a settlement conference before a judge, and failure to do so can result in sanctions.

New Hampshire – A hearing panel may commence prior to initiating litigation on a voluntary basis. The findings must be on a preponderance of the evidence, and can be admissible as evidence if the panel's decision was unanimous and the opposing party takes the case to trial.

New Mexico – A medical review commission evaluates all claims prior to filing a complaint. The decision is non-binding and inadmissible.

Utah – Voluntary pre-litigation panel is not admissible and nonbinding.

Virginia – Any party can request a review panel that consists of two attorneys. The opinion is nonbinding, admissible as evidence, but not conclusive.

Wyoming – All cases must be submitted to a pre-trial screening panel. The decision is by majority vote and is not binding. The decision may be admissible in a subsequent trial.

References

American Medical Association (AMA), *Select State Laws II, Liability Reform.pdf* February 2008, www.ama-assn.org

McCullough, Campbell & Lane LLP, *Summary of Medical Malpractice Law*, http://www.mcandl.com/states.html

American Tort Reform Association State and Federal Reforms, http://www.atra.org/reforms/

Expertlaw *Medical Malpractice Law – A State By State Overview*, http://www.expertlaw.com/library/malpractice_by_state/

Onecle Court Opinions, *Florida Torts Code Section 766.108*, http://law.onecle.com/florida/torts/766.108.html

South Carolina Legislature Online, Title 15, Section 15-79-120 and 15-79-125, http://www.scstatehouse.gov/code/t15c079.htm

Appendix C **Collateral source reform**

Collateral source: States typically ignore collateral sources of income or insurance when awarding damages to give a larger verdict. States that are listed as reforming the statute are assumed to have eliminated the rule unless otherwise indicated.

States that have reformed the Collateral Source rule

Alabama

Alaska – Exception does not include evidence of benefits received from a federal program that must subrogate (that is take action to recover the amount of a claim, if caused by a third party, by going after that party), or death benefits paid under a life insurance policy.

Arizona, California, Colorado

Connecticut – Plaintiff can use the amount of premiums paid to add to the economic damages.

Delaware – Only applicable for public sources of payments. Does not include evidence of benefits from life insurance or private collateral sources.

Florida – Exception if a right of subrogation exists.

Idaho – Exception for federal benefits, life insurance proceeds, or subrogation rights.

Illinois – If a defendant applies 30 days after judgment, award can be reduced: fifty percent of lost wages or disability income, one hundred percent of medical payments made by another entity. Exceptions for right of subrogation, and premium payments by claimant are added to judgment.

Indiana – Evidence of life insurance or other death benefits, benefits paid by claimant or family, or payments made by state or U.S. prior to trial are not considered collateral sources of payment.

How to Survive a Medical Malpractice Lawsuit. By © Ilene R. Brenner. Published 2010 Blackwell Publishing, ISBN: 978-1-4443-3130-1.

Iowa, Maine

Massachusetts – Deduction occurs post verdict, and exceptions for right of subrogation are made.

Michigan – Life insurance proceeds are excepted.

Minnesota – Exceptions for life insurance payments and premium payments by claimant.

Montana – Only in cases where damages exceed $50,000.

Nebraska – Exceptions for premium payments by claimant.

Nevada

New Jersey – Exceptions for worker's compensation and life insurance benefits.

New York – Reduction of damages shall be offset by premiums paid by the claimant for two years preceding the action and projected future cost of maintaining benefits.

North Dakota – Exceptions for life insurance, death or retirement benefits, or payments from insurance coverage purchased by the plaintiff.

Ohio – Exception for rights of subrogation.

Oklahoma – Exception for rights of subrogation.

Oregon – Exception for life insurance benefits for which the claimant has paid, retirement/disability, social security, or insurance benefits for which the person or deceased paid premiums.

Pennsylvania – Plaintiff cannot sue for damages that were paid by the health insurer.

Rhode Island

South Dakota – Exception for sources that are subject to subrogation, or purchased by the claimant.

Tennessee – Exception for private insurance or other benefits paid for by the plaintiff.

Utah – Exception for sources that are subject to subrogation, and amount paid to secure benefits.

Washington, West Virginia

States that continue to allow Collateral Sources

Arkansas, D.C.

Georgia – Laws that allowed a reduction of damages from collateral sources were declared unconstitutional.

Hawaii
Kansas – Laws that allowed a reduction of damages from collateral sources was declared unconstitutional.
Kentucky – Laws that allowed a reduction of damages from collateral sources was declared unconstitutional.
Louisiana, Maryland, Mississippi, Missouri
New Hampshire – Laws that allowed a reduction of damages from collateral sources was declared unconstitutional.
New Mexico, North Carolina, South Carolina, Texas, Vermont, Virginia]

References

American Medical Association (AMA), *Select State Laws II, Liability Reform.pdf*, February 2008, www.ama-assn.org

McCullough, Campbell & Lane LLP, *Summary of Medical Malpractice Law*, http://www.mcandl.com/states.html

American Tort Reform Association State and Federal Reforms, http://www.atra.org/reforms/

Expertlaw *Medical Malpractice Law – A State By State Overview*, http://www.expertlaw.com/library/malpractice_by_state/

Appendix D **I'm Sorry Laws**

I'm Sorry: Generally, these laws protect health care providers who express sympathy to a patient for an unanticipated outcome from having such statement used against the physician in a subsequent lawsuit. It is to encourage open communication between patients and physicians without fear of reprisal. The type of expressions covered by the law and their level of protection vary among the states. Some states only protect for expressions of sympathy, and some states protect for all admissions of fault.

States that protect for expressions of sympathy

The laws apply to any statements, gestures, or expressions of apology, benevolence, sympathy, or commiseration made by a health care provider to an alleged victim of an unanticipated outcome or the victim's relative or representative. Apology laws in these states protect any expressions of sympathy, condolence and regret, but not specific admissions of fault.

California, Delaware, Florida, Hawaii, Idaho, Illinois, Indiana, Iowa, Louisiana, Maine, Maryland, Massachusetts, Missouri, Montana, Nebraska, New Hampshire, North Carolina, North Dakota, Ohio, Oklahoma, Oregon, Rhode Island, South Dakoka, Tennessee, Texas, Utah, Virginia, West Virginia

States that protect all admissions of fault

Arizona, Colorado, Connecticut, Georgia, South Carolina, Vermont, Wyoming

States with individual statutes

District of Columbia – Applies to the use of expressions of sympathy or regret made in writing, orally, or by conduct to the injured patient, the patient's family, or anyone who claims damages through the victim.

How to Survive a Medical Malpractice Lawsuit. By © Ilene R. Brenner. Published 2010 Blackwell Publishing.

Hawaii – Applies to evidence of written or oral apologies and evidence of benevolent gestures made in connection with such apologies.

Illinois – Law is limited to expressions of grief, apology or explanation made within 72 hours of when the provider knew or should have known of the potential cause of such outcome.

Vermont – Only applies to oral expressions of regret or apology.

States with no protections for apologies

Alaska, Alabama, Arkansas, Kansas, Kentucky, Mississippi, Nevada, New Mexico, Pennsylvania, New Jersey, New York

References

American Medical Association (AMA), *I'm Sorry Laws, Summary of State Laws*, 11_2007_TheLaw_Chart1.pdf, February 2008, www.ama-assn.org

Sorry Works! Coalition (http://www.sorryworks.net/lawdoc.phtml); *Narrative Review: Do State Laws Make It Easier to Say "I'm Sorry".* Ann Intern Med 2008; 149: 811-815.

Glossary

Admission Against Interest: An admission of the truth of a fact by parties to a lawsuit, when a statement obviously would be against their personal interests.

Against Medical Advice (AMA) Form: A form found in many hospitals, which confirms that a patient is of their own volition leaving the care of the physician and hospital despite a medical necessity to stay. It is used to absolve the healthcare entity of liability; however, the form alone may not be sufficient.

Alternative Dispute Resolution (ADR): Any means of settling a legal claim outside of the courtroom.

Appeal: A request for a new hearing to a higher court on issues of law.

Appellate Court: A higher court with the jurisdiction to review the decision of a lower court.

Arbitration: A form of alternative dispute resolution, which is a non-court procedure for resolving legal disputes using a neutral third party as a arbitrator whereby the decision is binding.

Authoritative Source: A written document that sets the guidelines on a particular topic that is used to establish, along with expert testimony, the standard of care in a legal dispute. Physicians should never agree to any particular document as being authoritative. Textbooks and articles may record what should be standard care but are not the standard of care.

Bad Outcome: When a statistically probable adverse outcome occurs that did not occur as a result of any negligence on the physician's part.

Claim: An oral or written statement stating allegations of negligence against the physician in a malpractice case.

Claims-Made Policy: A claim (or potential claim) against the physician must be made during the insurance policy period. If a claim were to be made after the policy period, but occur during the policy period, the physician would not be covered for that claim.

How to Survive a Medical Malpractice Lawsuit. By © Ilene R. Brenner. Published 2010 Blackwell Publishing.

Closing Statements: Synonym of closing arguments/summation. After all the testimony and cross-examination has been completed, these are the final statements made by the attorney in front of the jury before the jury goes to deliberate, which must discuss the evidence and inferences of facts made in the course of the trial. The attorneys may not discuss issues outside of this case or about new evidence not presented at trial.

Co-Defendant: A defendant who has been joined together with at least one other defendant in a single lawsuit.

Collateral Sources: When a jury is determining the economic damages that a plaintiff incurred, any monies that a plaintiff receives from a source such as medicaid or an insurance policy who are not party to the lawsuit are considered collateral sources and depending on the state law may or may not be deducted from the economic damages the defendant has to pay.

Complaint: Written notice to the defendant that a legal action is underway. A written document that states negligence, proximate cause, and damages against a physician in a medical malpractice lawsuit—usually accompanied by a summons.

Conflict of Interest: A situation where the attorney has a duty to more than one defendant, but cannot adequately represent the actual or potential adversarial interests of both parties.

Consent to Settle: A clause in a physician's professional liability insurance policy giving the doctors the right to consent before the insurance company can settle their case.

Cross-Examination: The questioning of a witness at trial by the opposing party's attorney.

Damages: Monetary compensation that is awarded by the court or jury in a civil action.

Daubert Standard: Legal precedent set in 1993 by the Supreme Court of the United States in the case *Daubert v. Merrell Dow Pharmaceuticals* regarding the admissibility of novel scientific evidence and expert witness testimony during federal legal proceedings.

Defendant: The party against whom a lawsuit is filed.

Deliberation: When a jury considers the evidence and renders a verdict.

Deposition: One party before trial in a legal proceeding asks questions of a witness outside of a courtroom setting.

Directed Verdict: Where the plaintiffs fail in their burden of proof, on motion of the attorney representing the defendant, a judge can direct a verdict for the doctor.

Direct Examination: The questioning of witnesses at trial by the party that calls them to testify.

Discovery: Part of the pretrial process of requesting relevant information and documents from the other side, and includes interrogatories, requests for document production and depositions.

Duty: Legal obligation of a physician to care for the patient.

Economic Damages: Provide compensation for objectively verifiable monetary losses such as past and future medical expenses and loss of past and future earnings.

EMTALA: The Emergency Medical Treatment and Active Labor Act governs when and how a patient may be refused treatment or transferred to another hospital. The goal is to prevent hospitals from rejecting patients without insurance or ability to pay. If a medical screening exam determines that the patient does not have an emergency medical condition, the hospital has no further obligations.

Expert Witness: A person with special knowledge, training, or experience who states their opinion in court on the issues in the case despite not being present at the event. They are used to determine the standard of care in medical malpractice lawsuits.

Final Disposition (of the case): The final determination of a case in court.

HIPAA: The Health Insurance and Portability Accountability Act of 1996. There are two sections to the act. Title 1 concerns health insurance coverage for people who lose or change jobs. Title 2 seeks to establish standardized mechanisms for healthcare data confidentiality and security.

Hung Jury: When a jury is unable to come to a final decision leading to a mistrial and a new trial.

Indemnification: When one party is contractually obligated to guarantee against the loss of another party. In medical malpractice cases where there is an employer and employee relationship and there is vicarious liability, if there is a verdict over the employee's insurance limits, the employer must pay the overage of the employee's insurance, and in a separation action sue the employee to get back the overage that they were forced to pay.

Informed Consent: A procedure to ensure that a patient knows all of the risks involved in a treatment or procedure. The elements of informed consents include informing the patient of the nature of the treatment, possible alternative treatments, and the potential risks, complications, and benefits of the treatment. For informed consent to be considered valid, the patient must be competent and the consent given voluntarily.

Interrogatory: Written questions that are part of the pretrial discovery, asked of the plaintiffs and defendants by the opposing attorneys. Witnesses such as experts are not part of the interrogatory process; if questions are asked of them pretrial, it is through a deposition.

Judgment: A decision by the court resolving a lawsuit and specifying the rights and obligations of the parties. It is the court's official pronouncement of the law made in writing and stating the winner of the case and the damages owed.

Jury Charges: Jury instruction where the judge gives an explanation of the law involved in the case. These are given after the final arguments and before deliberations.

Jury Panel: The group of people who serve as the pool to select a jury.

Jury Selection: The process by which a jury is chosen.

Liability: Fault or departure in a medical malpractice case.

Mediation: Form of alternative dispute resolution where two parties try to resolve their legal differences outside of court using a neutral third party. However, it is different from arbitration in that a mediator has no power to impose a solution.

Medical Malpractice: Negligent treatment of a patient by a healthcare professional or organization.

Mid-Level Provider: Synonym with physician extender. Healthcare professional, either a physician's assistant or nurse practitioner who is trained in medicine but does not have the extensive training of a physician. They usually practice under the auspices of a physician; however, many states allow independent practice and prescription-writing ability.

Motion: A written or oral request made to a judge to obtain a favorable ruling.

National Practitioner Data Bank (NPDB): An alert or flagging system intended to facilitate a comprehensive review of healthcare practitioners' professional credentials. The information contained in the NPDB is intended to direct discrete inquiry into, and scrutiny of, specific areas of a practitioner's licensure, professional society memberships, medical malpractice payment history, and record of clinical privileges. Any entity that makes a payment on behalf of a physician (e.g., hospital or insurance carrier) in settlement of a written complaint or claim or judgment must report that payment info to the NPDB. In other words, any payment, for as low as one penny, is reportable once a written complaint or claim has been made. However, settlement payments that are made before a formal claim or demand has been made are not automatically reportable (e.g., money paid to patient for medical error to prevent them from suing).

Negligence: Breach of a duty of care that causes injury to another person.

Negotiation: It is a form of alternative dispute resolution whereby two or more parties confer together in good faith so as to settle a matter of mutual concern.

Noneconomic Damages: Damages that do not involve monetary concerns such as loss of wages and medical bills. Some examples include pain, suffering, loss of consortium, and loss of quality of life.

Notice of Appeal: A written document filed by the appellant (party making the appeal) with the court and notice given to the opposing party as the initial step in the appeal process. It informs the court and the party in whose favor a judgment has been made that the unsuccessful party seeks an appeal of the case.

Occurrence Policy: Medical malpractice insurance policy that covers a medical practitioner from any incident occurring while the policy is in force and covers those claims forever regardless of whether the physician still has that same policy.

Opening Statements: Statement made by the attorneys at the beginning of the trial. It outlines the evidence they intend to introduce to support their case.

Peer Review: Scrutiny by a physician's peers, also called quality assurance, and usually conducted by risk management. The issues discussed in this setting are protected from discovery and cannot be admitted as evidence. The aim is to raise the quality of care, reduce costs, avoid expensive litigation, enhance hospital reputation, and protect accreditation. Consequences of censure from a peer review include possible loss of credentials, suspension, or revocation of hospital privileges.

Physician Extender: Synonym with mid-level provider. Healthcare professional, either a physician's assistant or nurse practitioner who is trained in medicine but does not have the extensive training of a physician. They usually practice under the auspices of a physician; however, many states allow independent practice and prescription-writing ability.

Plaintiff: The person who initiates a lawsuit.

Preparation Expert: Person who gives advice to a party to prepare the party for deposition or trial.

Pretrial Screening Panel: A form of alternative dispute resolution whereby medical injury claims are evaluated to encourage the settlement of claims outside of a courtroom. Although (depending on the state) the decision of the panel may be admissible in court, the decision is not binding as it is in arbitration.

Process Server: A person legally authorized to deliver legal process, usually a subpoena or summons and complaint, to a witness or party to a lawsuit.

Proximate Cause: A critical element to prove medical negligence. It is defined legally as a causative element which, in a natural and continuous sequence, is unbroken by any intervening event, produces injury, and without which, the injury would not have occurred.

Punitive Damages: Damages that are not considered economic or non-economic, which are issued to punish a losing party for willful or malicious misconduct and act as a deterrent from committing similar acts in the future.

Re-Cross: In a trial, after the re-direct examination is completed, a follow-up cross-examination can occur to address issues that were brought up.

Re-Direct: In a trial, questioning a witness regarding issues that were brought up in the cross-examination.

Risk Management: A risk is an exposure to the possibility of injury or financial loss. Thus, risk management is the process by which liability is assessed and dealt with, which has three basic components—prevention of injury, financing for risks, and the management of claims. A comprehensive quality control program, for example, peer review, is essential to the process.

Rest: When a party in court indicates that no further evidence and testimony will be offered.

Settlement: Resolution of a claim by mutual agreement to avoid a trial.

Standard of Care: Good and accepted medical practice as established by experts in the course of a trial.

Statute of Limitations: The legally determined time limit by which a lawsuit must be filed.

Subpoena: An order of the court for a witness to appear at a particular time or place—or to produce documents that is under control of the witness.

Summation: Synonym of closing statements/arguments. After all the testimony and cross-examination has been completed, these are the final statements made by the attorney in front of the jury before the jury goes to deliberate, which may discuss the evidence and inferences from the facts made in the course of the trial. The attorneys may not discuss issues outside of this case or about new evidence not presented at trial. Plaintiff's attorney opens first and closes last.

Summons: The document that officially starts a lawsuit and tells the defendant they are being sued and commands them to answer the complaint made by the plaintiff.

Testimony: Oral evidence given under oath by a witness.

Verdict: The formal decision made by a jury concerning the questions raised at trial.

Vicarious Liability: This is a legal concept that imposes liability on one party for the actions of that party's agent. When an employer hires an employee, the employee is acting as an agent for the employer, and the employer is therefore liable for the employee's actions. In other words, you can be liable for the actions of your employees or partners.

Voir Dire: From old French, meaning "To speak the truth." It is the examination of a jury panel to determine their qualifications and suitability to sit on a jury.

Index

Printed in the USA/Agawam, MA
July 26, 2022

795867.019